AF616298

54027000427433

PHARMACEUTICAL TECHNOLOGY
Controlled Drug Release
Volume 2

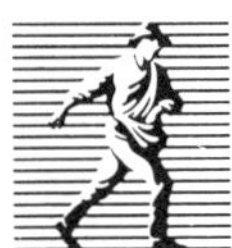

ELLIS HORWOOD SERIES IN PHARMACEUTICAL TECHNOLOGY

Editor: Professor M. H. RUBINSTEIN, School of Health Sciences, Liverpool Polytechnic

UNDERSTANDING EXPERIMENTAL DESIGN AND INTERPRETATION IN PHARMACEUTICS
N. A. Armstrong & K. C. James
MICROBIAL QUALITY ASSURANCE IN PHARMACEUTICALS, COSMETICS AND TOILETRIES
Edited by S. Bloomfield *et al.*
PHARMACEUTICAL PRODUCT LICENSING: Requirements for Europe
Edited by A. C. Cartwright & B. R. Matthews
DRUG DISCOVERY TECHNOLOGIES
C. Clark & W. H. Moos
PHARMACEUTICAL PRODUCTION FACILITIES: Design and Applications
G. Cole
PHARMACEUTICAL TABLET AND PELLET COATING
G. Cole
THE PHARMACY AND PHARMACOTHERAPY OF ASTHMA
Edited by P. F. D'Arcy & J. C. McElnay
GUIDE TO MICROBIOLOGICAL CONTROL IN PHARMACEUTICALS
Edited by S. P. Denyer & R. M. Baird
RECEPTOR DATA FOR BIOLOGICAL EXPERIMENTS: A Guide to Drug Selectivity
Edited by H. N. Doods and J. C. A. van Meel
PHARMACEUTICAL THERMAL ANALYSIS: Techniques and Applications
J. L. Ford and P. Timmins
PHYSICO-CHEMICAL PROPERTIES OF DRUGS: A Handbook for Pharmaceutical Scientists
P. Gould
DRUG DELIVERY TO THE GASTROINTESTINAL TRACT
Edited by J. G. Hardy, S. S. Davis and C. G. Wilson
POLYPEPTIDE AND PROTEIN DRUGS: Production, Characterization and Formulation
Edited by R. C. Hider and D. Barlow
HANDBOOK OF PHARMACOKINETICS: Toxicity Assessment of Chemicals
J. P. Labaune
TABLET MACHINE INSTRUMENTATION IN PHARMACEUTICS: Principles and Practice
P. Ridgway Watt
PHARMACEUTICAL CHEMISTRY, Volume 1 Drug Synthesis
H. J. Roth *et al.*
PHARMACEUTICAL CHEMISTRY, Volume 2 Drug Analysis
H. J. Roth *et al.*
PHARMACEUTICAL TECHNOLOGY: Controlled Drug Release, Volume 1
Edited by M. H. Rubinstein
PHARMACEUTICAL TECHNOLOGY: Controlled Drug Release, Volume 2
Edited by J. I. Wells and M. H. Rubinstein
PHARMACEUTICAL TECHNOLOGY: Tableting Technology, Volume 1
Edited by M. H. Rubinstein
PHARMACEUTICAL TECHNOLOGY: Tableting Technology, Volume 2
Edited by M. H. Rubinstein
PHARMACEUTICAL TECHNOLOGY: Drug Stability
Edited by M. H. Rubinstein
PHARMACEUTICAL TECHNOLOGY: Drug Targeting*
Edited by M. H. Rubinstein
UNDERSTANDING ANTIBACTERIAL ACTION AND RESISTANCE
A. D. Russell and I. Chopra
RADIOPHARMACEUTICALS USING RADIOACTIVE COMPOUNDS IN PHARMACEUTICS AND MEDICINE
Edited by A. Theobald
PHARMACEUTICAL PREFORMULATION: The Physicochemical Properties of Drug Substances
J. I. Wells
PHYSIOLOGICAL PHARMACEUTICS: Biological Barriers to Drug Absorption
C. G. Wilson & N. Washington
PHARMACOKINETIC MODELLING USING STELLA ON THE APPLE™ MACINTOSH™
C. Washington, N. Washington & C. Wilson

PHARMACEUTICAL TECHNOLOGY

Controlled Drug Release

Volume 2

Editors:

JAMES I. WELLS B.Sc., M.Sc., Ph.D., M.R.Pharm.S., M.Inst. Pkg.
Formulation Team Leader, Aston Molecules, Birmingham

MICHAEL H. RUBINSTEIN Ph.D., B.Pharm., C.Chem., M.R.Pharm.S.
Professor of Pharmaceutical Technology
School of Health Sciences, Liverpool Polytechnic

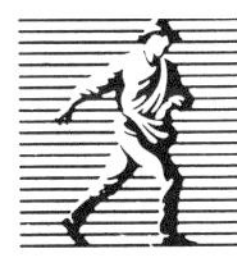

ELLIS HORWOOD
NEW YORK LONDON TORONTO SYDNEY TOKYO SINGAPORE

First published in 1991 by
ELLIS HORWOOD LIMITED
Market Cross House, Cooper Street,
Chichester, West Sussex, PO19 1EB, England

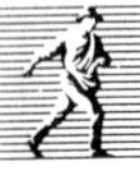

A division of
Simon & Schuster International Group
A Paramount Communications Company

Typeset in Times by Ellis Horwood Limited
Printed and bound in Great Britain
by Bookcraft Ltd, Midsomer Norton, Avon

British Library Cataloguing-in-Publication Data

Pharmaceutical technology: Vol. 2.
Controlled drug release. —
(Ellis Horwood series in pharmaceutical technology)
I. Wells, James, I. II. Rubinstein, Michael, H. III. Series
615
ISBN 0–13–662941–5

Library of Congress Cataloging-in-Publication Data available

Table of contents

Chapters 1, 4, 6, 7, 9, 10, 11, 14, 15 and 16 are from the 8th Pharmaceutical Technology Conference, Monte Carlo, 29–31 March, 1989.

Chapters 2, 3, 5, 8, 12, 13 and 17 are from the 9th Pharmaceutical Technology Conference, Veldhoven, The Netherlands, 4–6 April, 1990.

Preface

This book is a companion volume to *Pharmaceutical Technology: Controlled Drug Release*, Volume 1, edited by M. H. Rubinstein and published in 1987. It focused on the different types of polymeric materials used in controlled release. This book extends these concepts to include drug properties, design and optimization, coating, the effect of food and pharmacokinetics. It also reflects the growing interest in biodegradable polymers in oral and topical formulations and the use of sterile implants.

The chapters are selected from the papers presented at two Pharmaceutical Technology Conferences: Monte Carlo in 1989 and Veldhoven, The Netherlands, in 1990 and reflect the current state of the art. Chapters 1–8 deal with matrix systems and 9 to 11 with multiparticulate formulations. Chapters 12, 13 and 14 examine opportunities with biodegradable polymers. While the oral route remains the major application, topical (Chapter 8), ophthalmics (Chapters 15–16) and implants (Chapters 16 and 17) are also discussed.

While new drugs continue to possess advantageous therapeutic profiles but poor pharmacokinetics with short half-lives, controlled release will continue to demand pharmaceutical skill. The increasing number of biological peptide drugs will increase this demand still further. This book will provide a wide-ranging cornucopia from which experience and new ideas can be distilled. Indeed:

A little of what you fancy does you good.
Marie Lloyd 1870–1922

Cotherstone
May 1991

James I. Wells

Slow and steady wins the race

Poems. The Hare and the Tortoise.
Robert Lloyd 1733–1764

Matrix formulations

1

Influence of drug solubility in the formulation of hydrophilic matrices

B. Huet de Barochez, J. S. Julien, F. Lapeyre, S. Horvath and **A. Cuiné**
Ardix, 25 rue E. Vignat, F-45000 Orléans, France

INTRODUCTION

Sustained release dosage forms are a convenient means to obtain a reduction in daily administration of drugs with fast absorption and/or elimination. In this study three different drugs are compared: one is slightly water soluble, and two are highly water soluble (Table 1). Production of hydrophilic matrices is a well-known technology, by direct compression as well as by wet granulation [1,2]. A lot of research has been done and the literature on this subject is plentiful. Different polymers may be used to control the diffusion of the drug. Among them, hydroxypropylmethylcellulose (HPMC) seems most employed [3–5].

Table 1 — Drug characteristics

	Drug A	Drug B	Drug C
Solubility in water	about 0.5%	>50%	>50%
pK_a	—	4.0, 9.0	8
Half-live (plasma)	<12 h	<6 h	<8 h

MATERIALS

The following ingredients were used for the preparation of hydrophilic matrices: calcium hydrogen phosphate dihydrate, (SPCI, La Plaine Saint Denis), calcium hydrogen phosphate for direct compression (Emcompress, SPCI), lactose 150 mesh (Sucre de Lait, Sains-du-Nord), lactose Fast Flo (SEPPIC, Paris), polyvinylpyrrolidone (PVP) (Luviscol K30, BASF, Levallois), HPMC (Methocel K4M and E4M CR, Colorcon, Bougival or Metolose 60SH4000 and 90SH4000, SEPPIC), hydroxyethylcellulose (HEC) (Natrosol, Aqualon, Rueil-Malmaison), magnesium stearate (Stéarinerie Dubois, Paris) and colloidal silicon dioxide (Aerosil 200, Degussa, Neuilly sur Seine).

Different grades of Methocel and Metolose are supplied, with nominal viscosities of 4000 mPa s (measured with a Brookfield viscometer on a 2% w/v solution). Methocel 4M types E and K are different in their hydration rates, type K being the quickest. Metoloses SH4000 differ in their gel temperature. Grades 60 and 90 were used. Another polymer of 4000 mPa s viscosity was used: hydroxyethylcellulose, in order to observe effects on the dissolution rate.

FORMULATION, PREPARATION AND TESTS

Drug A

With drug A, HPMC was used at different concentrations, from 25.3% to 41.0% (Table 2). Five 1 kg batches were prepared using direct compression. Lactose and Emcompress were mixed together, using a rotary mixer, and then drug was incorporated by trituration. HPMC was mixed with Aerosil 200 in the same mixer, blended with the first mix, mixed and lubricated with magnesium stearate. Compression was conducted on a MR12 rotary press (Frogerais, Ivry sur Seine) equipped with 7 mm diameter punches with a 5 mm concavity. Compression force was adjusted to obtain tablets with a hardness of about 7 daN.

Table 2 — DC tablet formulae (mg)

	1	2	3	4	5
Drug A	3.0	3.0	3.0	3.0	3.0
HPMC	40.0	50.0	60.0	70.0	82.0
Fast Flo lactose	42.6	42.6	42.6	42.6	42.6
Emcompress	71.0	71.0	71.0	71.0	71.0
Aerosil 200	0.4	0.4	0.4	0.4	0.4
Magnesium stearate	1.0	1.0	1.0	1.0	1.0

Two batches were prepared by wet granulation, one with lactose as a diluent (Table 3), the other with calcium hydrogen phosphate. Diluent, drug and PVP were mixed together at 200 rev min^{-1} in a high speed granulator dryer (Turbo-sphère) TS10 (Moritz, Chatou). The mixture was granulated at the same speed for 5 min, using a 30–70 water–alcohol solution. After drying (60°C under vacuum), the

Table 3 — Wet massed tablet formulae (mg)

	6	7
Drug A	2.5	2.5
Lactose	114.9	—
Calcium hydrogen phosphate	—	114.9
PVP	6.2	6.2
HPMC	74.0	74.0
Aerosil 200	0.4	0.4
Magnesium stearate	2.0	2.0

product was sized with an oscillating granulator, blended with HPMC in a rotary mixer, then lubricated with Aerosil and magnesium stearate in the same mixer. Compression was conducted on a rotary press (MR12) equipped with 8 mm diameter punches with 7 mm concavity.

A third batch was prepared with formula 6, using a planetary mixer for the granulation. It was dried in a ventilated oven.

Drug B

Formulae are described in Table 4. 6 kg batches of formulae 8–13 were prepared.

Table 4 — Tablet formulae (drug B)(mg)

	8	9	10	11	12	13
Drug B	80.00	40.00	40.00	40.00	80.00	80.00
Calcium hydrogen phosphate	92.00	46.00	46.00	112.00	92.00	221.00
PVP	13.30	6.65	6.65	13.30	13.30	16.20
HPMC	112.00	56.00	115.45	112.00	—	325.00
HEC	—	—	—	—	112.00	—
Aerosil 200	0.50	0.25	0.40	0.50	0.50	1.30
Magnesium stearate	2.20	1.10	1.50	2.20	2.20	6.50
Total	300.00	150.00	210.00	280.00	300.00	650.00
Punch diameter (mm)	9	7	8	9	9	12.5
Concavity (mm)	7	5	7	7	7	11

Calcium hydrogen phosphate was mixed for 5 min with drug and PVP at rev min^{-1} in a Moritz TS10. The mixture was granulated at the same speed for 5 min, after addition of a 30–70 (by volume) water–alcohol solution. After drying (60°C under vacuum), the product was sized with an oscillating granulator, blended for 10 min with HPMC or HEC in a rotary mixer, and then lubricant was added and mixed for 10 min in the same mixer. Compression was conducted on a rotary press (MR12).

Drug C

Formulations are described in Table 5. Mixing and granulation were carried out in a planetary mixer. After drying (60°C in a ventilated oven), the granulates were sized with an oscillating granulator, blended with HPMC and lubricants and compressed in order to obtain tablets of hardness about 6 daN.

Table 5 — Tablet formulae (drug C) (mg)

	14	15	16
Drug C	100.0	100.0	100.0
Calcium hydrogen phosphate	72.0	72.0	72.0
PVP	13.3	13.3	13.3
HPMC	112.0	161.5	211.0
Aerosil 200	0.5	0.6	0.7
Magnesium stearate	2.2	2.6	3.0
Total	300.0	350.0	400.0

Dissolution test

The dissolution test was carried out using the European Pharmacopoeia apparatus at a paddle speed of 100 rev min^{-1}. The dissolution medium was 900 ml of hydrochloric acid (0.05 N) (pH 1.6). Temperature was maintained at 37°C (±0.5°C). Samples of 10 ml were automatically withdrawn, filtered and analysed by UV spectophotometry. Four or six samples were analysed for each test. A study was conducted to assess the dependence of the dissolution rate on the pH: tests were conducted comparatively at pH 2, 5 and 7.4 with drug A and at pH 1.6 and 6.8 with drug B.

For non-linear dissolutions, values were fitted with equation (1) using non-linear regression with RS/1 software (BBN Software Product Corporation, Cambridge, MA):

$$y=100\,[1-\exp(-kt)] \quad (1)$$

In the case of linear dissolution, it follows equation (2):

$$y=kt \quad (2)$$

where y is the percentage of drug released at time t, k is a constant, characterizing the dissolution, and t is the time.

The t_{50} value was calculated from these equations (t_{50} represents the time for 50% drug release).

RESULTS AND DISCUSSION

Drug A

For direct compression, the dissolution rate is relatively dependent on the amount of HPMC. t_{50} varies from 4.75 h with 29.8% of HPMC to 12.25 h with 41.0% (Fig. 1). The dissolution rate follows zero-order release from 0% to 70%. In this case, dissolution is limited by the solubility of the drug in the matrix.

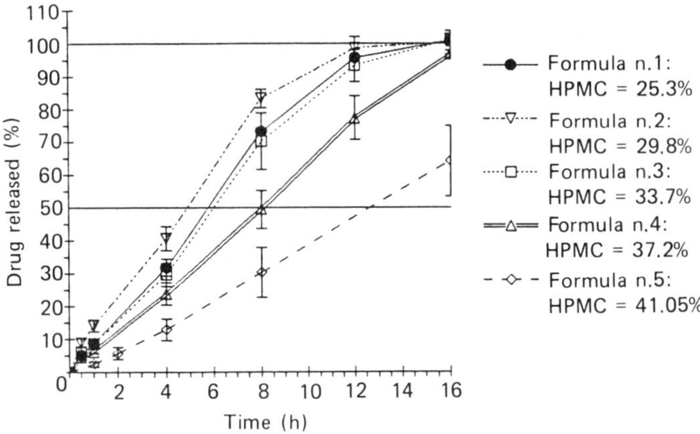

Fig. 1 — Effect of amount of HPMC on drug release for drug A.

The dissolution rate is very dependent on pH variations: with formula (41.0% HPMC), t_{50} increases from 10.0 h (pH 2.0) to 22.2 h (pH 7.4) (Fig. 2).

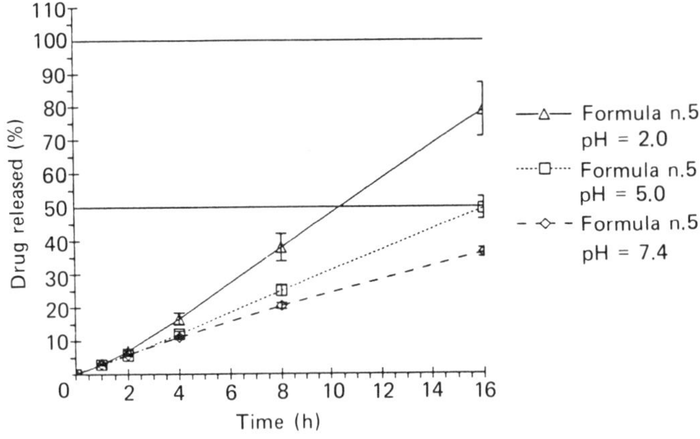

Fig. 2 — Effect of pH for drug A.

When tablets are prepared by wet granulation, the standard deviation of the dissolution rates seems to be dependent on the grain size distribution (Fig. 3). Mean

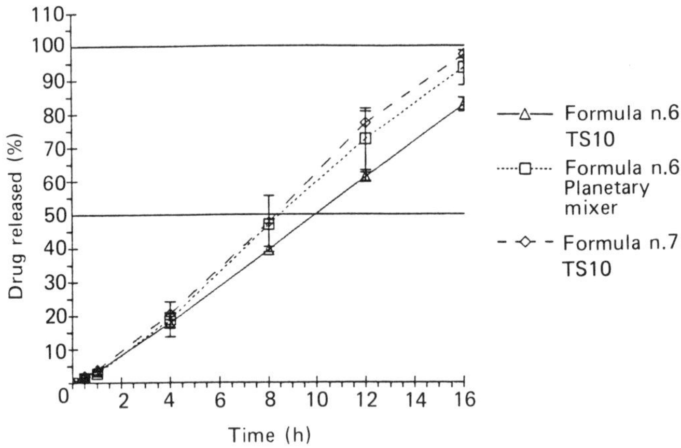

Fig. 3 — Effect of grain size for drug A.

diameters of batches prepared with the Moritz TS10 are 166 μm (formula 6) and 152 μm (formula 7). For the granulate prepared with a planetary mixer, the mean diameter is 326 μm and the distribution is wider (80% between 180 and 500 μm).

If calcium hydrogen phosphate is the only diluent, the dissolution rate is more dependent on pH variations (Fig. 4) than with lactose: t_{50} increases from 8.0 h (pH 2.0) to 22.1 h (pH 7.4) with calcium hydrogen phosphate, and from 9.7 h (pH 2.0) to 13.7 h (pH 7.4) with lactose.

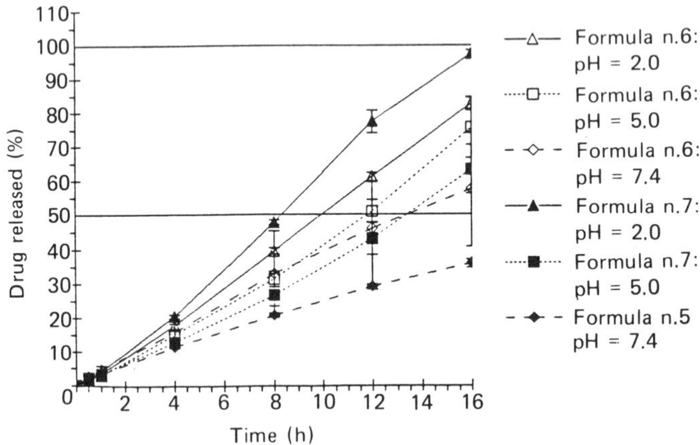

Fig. 4 — Effect of pH for drug A.

Drug B

The dissolution rate does not exhibit significant differences between Methocel E4M CR, Methocel K4M and Metolose 60SH4000 (formula 8): the respective t_{50} values are 1.78 h, 1.86 h and 1.75 h. Dissolution speed is higher with Metolose 90SH4000 (t_{50}=1.06 h) (Fig. 5) and Natrosol (formula 12: t_{50}=1.18 h) (Fig. 6). Standard

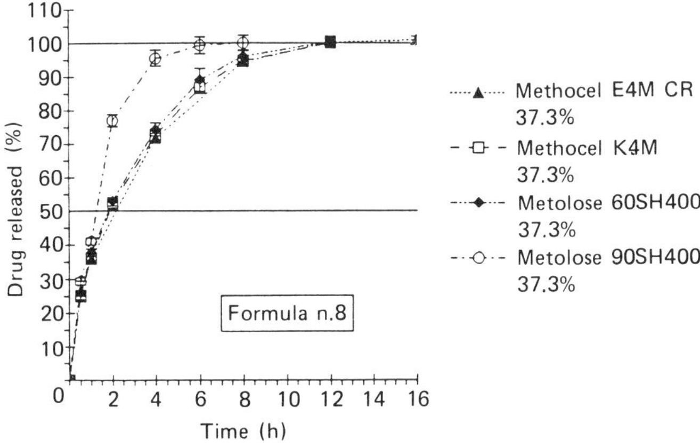

Fig. 5 — Drug release for formula 8.

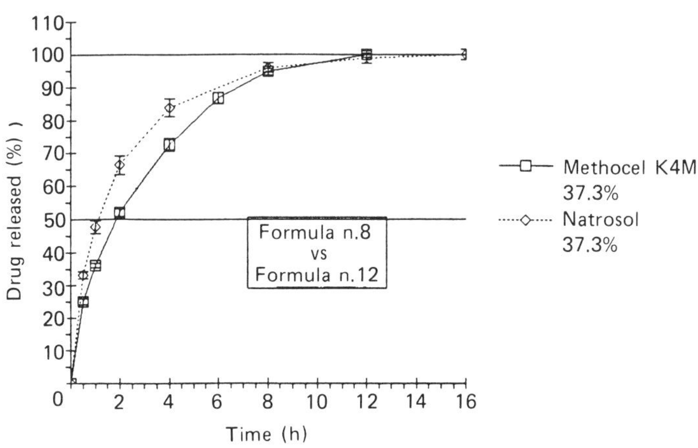

Fig. 6 — Drug release for formulae 8 and 12.

deviations are very low in all tests (<2%). pH variation has no effect on dissolution rate (Fig. 7).

If the same formula is compressed to half of the weight (formula 9 vs. formula 8), the dissolution rate increases (t_{50}=1.78 h for formula 8, t_{50}=1.15 h for formula 9). There are two ways to reduce this dissolution rate: (1) increasing the amount

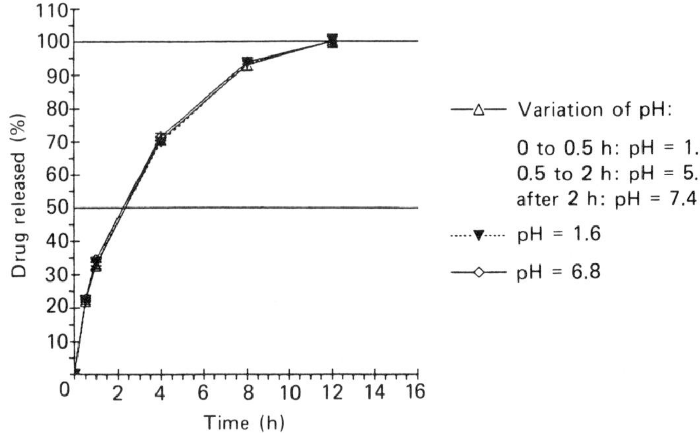

Fig. 7 — Effect of pH for drug B.

of HPMC by about 100% (formula 10, t_{50}=1.46 h), but, with such an augmentation, the dissolution rate does not increase very much, and compression is more difficult; (2) increasing the amount of calcium hydrogen phosphate in the granulate, before addition of HPMC and lubricants (formula 11, t_{50}=1.93 h).

If the quantity of HPMC is increased by threefold (formula 13), the quantity of calcium hydrogen phosphate must be augmented to obtain a compressible granulate. In this case, dissolution is only slightly reduced (t_{50}=2.50 h, Fig. 8).

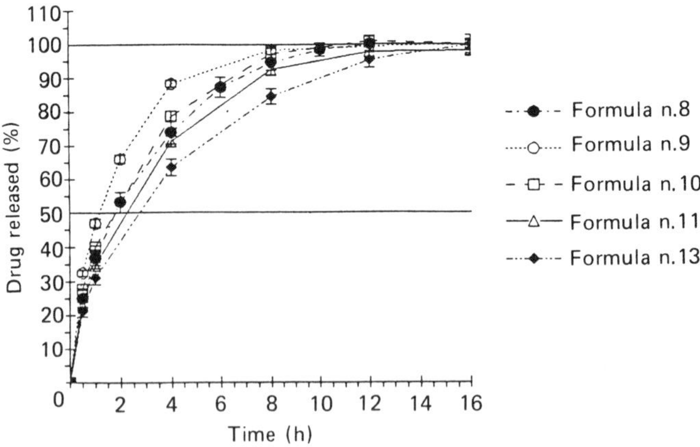

Fig. 8 — Effect of amount of HPMC on drug release for drug B.

Drug C

The physical characteristics of this drug are similar to those of drug B; dissolution rates are also similar with the same quantity of HMPC (formula 14: t_{50}=2.16 h). When the amount of HPMC is increased, the dissolution rate decreases, but slowly (Fig. 9).

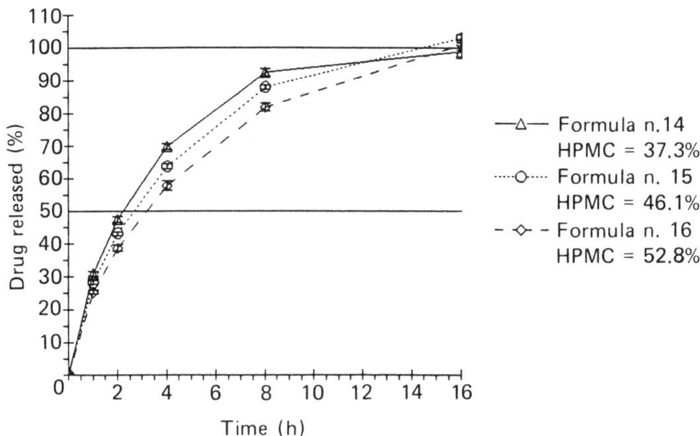

Fig. 9 — Effect of amount of HPMC on drug release for drug C.

CONCLUSION

Formulation of hydrophilic matrices with a release time longer than 8 h is difficult with drugs B and C, owing to the high solubility of the substances; contrary to slightly soluble drugs (e.g. drug A), zero-order release cannot be obtained by classical means. However, in this case, the dissolution rate is more sensitive to the quantities of hydrophilic polymer present, fabrication process, nature of the diluent and/or pH variations in the dissolution medium.

REFERENCES

[1] B. Huet de Barochez, F. Lapeyre and A. Cuinné, Oral sustained release dosage forms. Comparison between matrices and reservoir devices, *4th Int. Pharmaceutical Technology Symp., Ankara, 12–14, September 1988.*

[2] S. Segot-Chicq, E. Teillaud and N. A. Peppas, Les dispositifs à libération contrôlée pour la délivrance des principes actifs médicamenteux. I. Intérêt et applications, *STP Pharm*, **1** (1), 25–36 (1985).

[3] J. L. Avan and C. Brossard, Mise au point et développement technologique de matrices hydrophiles par compression directe sur machine rotative, *STP Pharma,* **1** (6), 516–622 (1985).

[4] J. L. Ford, M. H. Rubinstein and F. McCaul, Importance of drug type, tablet shape and formulation on release from hydroxypropylmethylcellulose matrix tables, *Proc. 6th Pharmaceutical Technology Conf. Canterbury, 7–9 April, 1987,* Vol. 1, pp. 82–87.

[5] P. Catellani, G. Vaona, P. Plazzi and P. Colombo, Compressed matrices: formulation and drug release kinetics, *Acta Pharm. Technol.,* **34** (1), 38–41 (1988).

[6] N. A. Peppas and S. Segot-Chico, Les dispositifs à libération contrôlèe pour la délivrance des principes actifs médicamenteux. III. Modélisation des mécanismes diffusionnels, *STP Pharma,* **1** (3), 208–216 (1985).

2

The effect of electrolytes and drugs on the cloud point of hydroxypropylmethylcellulose gels and the dissolution of drugs from hydroxypropylmethylcellulose matrix tablets

Karen Mitchell, James L. Ford†, David J. Armstrong, Peter N. C. Elliott and **Christopher Rostron**
The Drug Targeting Research Group, Centre for Pharmaceutical Sciences, School of Health Sciences, The Liverpool Polytechnic, Byrom Street, Liverpool L3 3AF, UK and
John E. Hogan
Colorcon Ltd, St. Paul's Cray, Orpington, Kent, UK

INTRODUCTION

Hydroxypropylmethylcellulose (HPMC) is used in dosage forms to provide sustained release. Relationships between drug release rates and formulation factors such as drug:HPMC ratio, viscosity grade, particle size of drug, added lubricant, added excipients, drug solubility and tablet shape have been evaluated using water as the dissolution media [1–3]. The hydration of HPMC is affected by temperature. As the gel temperature approaches, HPMC loses its water of hydration: this is accompanied by a drop in relative viscosity. As the polymer loses more water of hydration a polymer–polymer interaction takes place [4], giving a dramatic increase in relative viscosity, known as the gel point. Another phenomenon observed in HPMC gels with increase in temperature is a precipitation of the polymer; the developing turbidity may be measured by light transmission. The temperature at which light transmission reaches 50% is called the cloud point. The relationship between the thermal gelation temperature and the cloud point is complex: at low HPMC concentrations turbidity occurs before gelation occurs while at higher concentrations a gel is produced before turbidity is apparent. Both properties are similarly affected by electrolytes, i.e. one that reduces the cloud point will reduce the thermal gelation temperature [4]. Data

† Author to whom correspondence should be addressed.

on the effects of electrolytes on the thermal gelation temperature or cloud point of HPMC are limited [5].

This paper reports the effect of pH, electrolytes and drugs on the cloud points of HPMC gels and the effect of these electrolytes on the dissolution of propranolol hydrochloride from HPMC matrices and on the disintegration of HPMC matrices containing no drug.

MATERIALS AND METHODS

The HPMC was manufactured by Dow Chemicals (USA) as Methocel K15M and Methocel K100 grades. All solutes were of laboratory reagent standard obtained from British Drug Houses (Poole, UK) and all drugs were BP standard or better.

Cloud point studies

Quantities of gel (50 g) were prepared to contain 2% HPMC by dispersing the polymer into approximately 33% of the total weight of distilled water previously heated to 80°C, adding the required electrolyte or drug dissolved in distilled water and making up to weight. The gels were stored overnight to hydrate fully. Samples for analysis were transferred to disposable 1 cm^2 cuvettes and any air bubbles were removed by centrifugation. Samples were slowly heated and readings taken, initially at 5°C intervals but reducing to 1°C increments near the cloud points. The samples were measured spectrophotometrically at 800 nm against a 2% aqueous solution of the gel. For studies on the effect of pH on the cloud point gels were prepared without added electrolyte. Their pH was adjusted with 1 M HCl or 1 M NaOH following overnight hydration.

Disintegration studies

Shallow convex tablets ($\frac{1}{4}$ in) containing 300 mg HPMC K15M and 1% magnesium stearate were prepared by direct compression. Disintegration tests were performed in triplicate, using the BP 1988 method, in 600 ml of media at 37°C using discs. Tests were run for a maximum of 2 h.

Dissolution studies

Shallow convex tablets ($\frac{1}{4}$ in) containing 160 mg propranolol hydrochloride, 140 mg HPMC K15M and 1% magnesium stearate were prepared by direct compression. Three tablets were tested into 1 l of dissolution fluid buffer at 37°C using the British Pharmacopoeia (1988) basket method, rotating at 100 rev min^{-1} and monitoring propranolol at 288 nm. All media were prepared in molar concentrations and contained only the electrolyte stated. When the pH of the media was adjusted to pH 6 ± 0.2 either 1 M HCl or 1 M NaOH was used which did not significantly increase the ionic strength of the media.

The ionic strengths, I, of the solutions used for cloud point, disintegration and dissolution fluids were calculated according to equation (1):

$$I = 0.5 \sum (mz_2) \qquad (1)$$

where m is the molarity and z is the valence of each ion in the solution. Differences between molarity were considered to be too small to be significant.

RESULTS AND DISCUSSION

Effect of pH on cloud points

Although HPMC is not thought itself to be pH sensitive [6], the pH of a dissolution fluid is known to affect release rates of drugs from its matrices via the suppression of ionization [7]. The cloud points at 2% K100 gels (Table 1) were only affected by pH at low pHs. It was therefore considered unnecessary to modify the pH of electrolyte solutions used to determine cloud points.

Table 1 — The effect of pH on the cloud point of 2% K100 gels

Gel pH	Cloud point (°C)
1	64.5
3	68.8
5	70.5
7	70.5
9	70.5
12.23	69.7
K100 unadjusted	70.4

The effect of inorganic salts and drugs on the cloud point of 2% HPMC gels

Fig. 1 gives typical data. As the ionic strength of a particular electrolyte increased, the cloud point deceased (Tables 2 and 3). The ability of an electrolyte to salt out a polymer from its solution generally followed the salts' order in the lyotropic series. The relation between cloud point reduction and concentration of salt is generally thought to be linear but the relation is probably more complicated. At the low concentration of 0.02 M both drugs and electrolytes generally lowered the cloud point but at higher concentrations the drugs tended to raise the cloud point while the salts lowered it.

The cloud point may be regarded as a limit of solubility, since the turbidity produced is due to HPMC precipitating from solution. Equation (2) was used to determine the effect of salt concentration on the cloud point. Thus,

$$\log \mathrm{CP} = \log \mathrm{CP}_0 \pm K_{\mathrm{CP}} m \qquad (2)$$

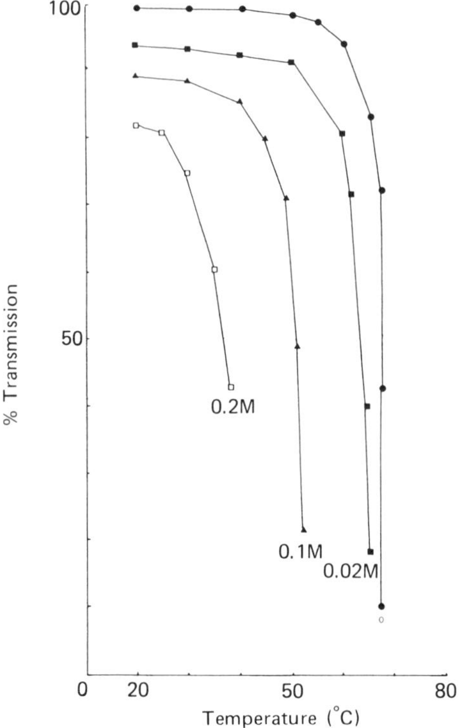

Fig. 1 — The effect of temperature on the light transmission of 2% HPMC K15M gels in water containing Na_2HPO_4.

where log CP is the observed cloud point of HPMC in the solution of the electrolyte, log CP_0 is a theoretical cloud point based on the intercept at zero solute concentration, K_{CP} is a salting-out constant analogous to that in equation (2) and m is the molal concentration. The gradient of the straight line, K_{CP}, is positive for 'salting in' and negative for 'salting out'. Values calculated by linear regression are given in Tables 2 and 3 respectively. It can be seen that the various sodium phosphate salts rank as tetrasodium pyrophosphate>trisodium orthophosphate>disodium hydrogen orthophosphate>sodium dihydrogen orthophosphate in order of their salting-out ability. The decrease in cloud point increased as the valence of the phosphate ion increased. However, in terms of ionic strength, sodium dihydrogen orthophosphate, the univalent salt, gave the greatest reduction. Additionally, the sodium salts more readily caused salting out than their corresponding potassium salts. The anions played a more significant role in determining cloud point reduction than cations; cf. Al^{3+} and Na^+.

The cloud points involving HPMC K15M gels were lower than those of HPMC K100 gels, a difference of ~2°C being noted. Sarkar [4] found ~6°C differences between the cloud points of 2% HPMC K100 and 2% HPMC K4M gels.

Table 2 — The effect of additives on the cloud points of 2% HPMC K100 gels

Additive	Concentration (molal) (unless otherwise stated)	Cloud point (°C)	*K*s	Correlation coefficient
None		70.4		
NaH_2PO_4	0.02	67.9		
	0.1	60.4	−0.63	0.9999
	0.2	52.3		
KH_2PO_4	0.02	66.4		
	0.1	60.0	−0.57	0.9998
	0.2	52.5		
Na_2HPO_4	0.02	66.5		
	0.1	51.7	−1.30	0.9997
	0.2	38.7		
Na_3PO_4	0.02	62.0		
	0.1	42.8	−2.20	0.9991
	0.2	25.0		
$Na_4P_2O_7$	0.02	60.7		
	0.1	39.0	−2.68	0.9969
	0.15	27.0		
K_2HPO_4	0.02	67.5		
	0.1	54.0	−1.20	0.9999
	0.2	41.0		
$AlCl_3$	0.02	70.4		
	0.1	66.4	−0.30	0.9995
	0.2	62.2		
NaCl	0.1	66.5		
	0.2	62.5		
	0.3	59.5	−0.22	0.9997
	0.5	54.0		
	1.0	41.5		
KCl	0.2	65.2		
	0.4	63.0	−0.10	0.9920
	0.6	59.7		
Potassium tartrate	0.02	66.3		
	0.1	54.0	−1.16	0.9998
	0.2	41.0		
Na_2SO_4	0.02	64.5		
	0.1	52.5	−1.28	0.9980
	0.2	38.0		
PEG 400	5%	75.0		
	10%	77.8	0.123	0.9998
	15%	80.5		
PEG 6000	5%	69.5		
	10%	66.6	−7.41	0.927
	15%	52.3		
Sodium lauryl sulphate	2%	>84.0		
	5%	>84.0		
	10%	>10%		

Touitou and Donbrow [8] noted that large ions, e.g. tetracaine hydrochloride, sodium salicylate and sodium benzoate, each with low affinities for water, raised the gelation temperature of HPMC. The effect is explained on the basis that a large ion is adsorbed onto the macromolecule, carrying with it water molecules raising the degree of hydration of the colloid. Quinine bisulphate, in spite of being water soluble and containing sulphate ions, did not affect the cloud point. One explanation could

Table 3 — The effect of additives on the cloud points of 2% HPMC K15M gels

Additives	Concentration (molal)	Cloud point (°C)	*K*s	Correlation coefficient
None		68.2		
NaH_2PO_4	0.02	64.5		
	0.1	59.5	−0.53	0.9962
	0.2	51.8		
Na_2HPO_4	0.02	63.8		
	0.1	50.5	−1.32	0.9998
	0.2	37.0		
Na_2PO_4	0.02	62.5		
	0.1	44.0	−2.32	0.9961
	0.2	24.0		
$Na_4P_2O_7$	0.02	60.5		
	0.06	49.5	−2.52	0.9969
	0.1	38.0		
Theophylline	0.02	67.5		
	0.075	66.5	0.00	
	0.1	66.5		
Propranolol HCl	0.02	67.5		
	0.1	71.0		
	0.2	82.0		
Aminophylline	0.02	68.0		
	0.1	72.5	0.32	0.9993
	0.2	77.8		
Promethazine HCl	0.02	65.5		
	0.05	65.5		
	0.09	66.0		
	0.2	>83.0		
Tetracycline HCl	0.02	67.4		
	0.1	71.3	0.35	0.9977
	0.2	78.0		
Quinine bisulphate	0.02	67.7		
	0.1	67.7	0.00	
	0.2	67.7		

be that the hydrating effect of the quinine molecule was counteracted by the dehydrating effect of the sulphate ion (Table 2). The poorly water-soluble theophylline did not affect the cloud point.

Aminophylline and tetracycline hydrochloride gave straight line relationships between their concentration in gels and the observed cloud points. In the case of tetracycline this did not explain a non-Higuchian release pattern previously found during dissolution from tetracyline–HPMC matrix tablets which was thought to be caused by a complex drug–HPMC gel interaction [3].

Propranolol hydrochloride and promethazine hydrochloride increased the gel points and no straight line relationship existed, indicating that at higher concentrations these drugs enable the polymer to hydrate to a much larger extent than at lower concentrations. Promethazine forms micelles at concentrations>0.5% w/v [9], which may be responsible for this behaviour. No critical micellar concentration is known for propanolol hydrochloride but from studies performed it is weakly surface active. The response of HPMC to these drugs may be associated with this surface activity.

Compounds including ethanol and polyethylene glycol increase the gel point by what is thought to be absorption of the large ion of relatively low water affinity onto the macromolecule [10], carrying with it water molecules and raising the degree of hydration [11]. However, differences were found between PEG 400 and PEG 6000 (Table 2) which caused salting in and out respectively, indicating a molecular weight dependence for PEG on the cloud point. The anionic surfactant sodium lauryl sulphate caused a salting in of the HPMC K100, probably by mechanisms similar to those of propanolol hydrochloride and promethazine hydrochloride.

The effect of salts on the disintegration of tablets

Touitou and Donbrow [8] have described three different kinds of responses when matrices were exposed to fluids containing solutes, namely (a) rapid disintegration, (b) gradual attrition and (c) maintenance of integrity. In Table 4 three different responses are shown to occur when HPMC K15M matrices without drug were exposed to disintegration tests. At low ionic strengths the matrices were unaffected by electrolytes and hydration occurred to produce an intact gel layer. At intermediate ionic strengths the matrices lost shape and integrity and disintegrated rapidly. The released particles did, however, slowly gel, indicating that hydration had not been prevented but merely retarded. This demonstrates how essential the rapid

Table 4 — The effect of solutes and ionic strength on disintegration times of HPMC K15M tablets

Additives	Concentration (M)	Ionic strength	Time (min)	Cloud point (°C)[a]	Matrix type[b]
NaH_2PO_4	0.9	0.9	52	18.9	2
	0.6	0.6	>120	29.2	1
KH_2PO_4	0.9	0.9	35	21.0	2
Na_2HPO_4	0.3	0.9	23	28.5	2
	0.8	2.4	>120	6.3	3
	0.1	0.3	>120	52.0	1
K_2HPO_4	0.3	0.9	18	31.0	2
NaCl	0.9	0.9	>120	43.7	1
	1.5	1.5	>120	32.0	1
	2.0	2.0	85	24.7	2
	2.5	2.5	>120	19.0	3
KCl	2.0	2.0	98	43.9	2
$AlCl_3$	0.35	2.1	>120	56.0	1
Na_2SO_4	0.3	0.9	35	28.5	2
K_2SO_4	0.3	0.9	24	—	2

[a] Cloud points based on K100 gels, not K15M.
[b] 1, rapid gelling, matrix intact; 2, slowly gelling, disintegration; 3, non-gelling.

production of a gel around a tablet is in maintaining the integrity of the matrix. At higher ionic strengths the matrices maintained their integrity, swelling slightly but not gelling. The matrix surface becomes porous, giving it a spongy texture. The ionic strengths which caused disintegration varied according to the salt used. Thus an ionic strength of 0.9 of sodium dihydrogen orthophosphate caused disintegration of the matrices within 1 h but a strength of 2.0 of sodium chloride was required to effect disintegration. Since the disintegration of the tablets can be explained by the salts decreasing the cloud point then their efffect on disintegration should also follow the lyotropic series. On this basis sodium salts appear anomalous since they should produce lower disintegration times than potassium salts. In studies on the disintegration of HPMC matrices, Fagan *et al.* [5] introduced a concept of threshold ionic strengths, where a matrix is not susceptible to ionic strengths below a certain point. This theory is not upheld by Table 4 which show that an ionic strength of 0.9, although resulting in disintegration of the matrices in solutions containing several of the salts, failed to facilitate disintegration when sodium chloride was used. Consequently disintegration depends on the susceptibility to the dehydration effects of specific ions rather than to a specific ionic strength.

The effect of salts on the dissolution of propanolol from HPMC K15M matrices

Since salts modified the disintegration of HPMC K15M matrices, dissolution from HPMC K15M matrices of propanolol hydrochloride was completed in order to determine salt effect on dissolution rate. Dissolution from matrices into media which had not been pH adjusted gave non-linear $t^{\frac{1}{2}}$ plots, e.g. in media containing disodium hydrogen orthophosphate or trisodium orthophosphate, indicating that precipitation of propanolol at the surface of the matrix occurred as a result of pH effects similar to those reported for promethazine hydrochloride [7]. Subsequent studies were performed in solutions at pH 6.0±0.2.

Drug release profiles from the tablets in various dissolution media are shown in Fig. 2. In all cases the release rates decreased initially from the control (distilled water) as electrolyte concentration increased, until a minimum release rate was obtained. As the electrolyte concentration further increased the release rates similarly increased until a 'burst' release occurred. These initial decreases in release rates were probably coincident with a decrease in polymer solubility, in that as the ionic strength of the dissolution medium is increased the cloud point is lowered towards 37°C. It may be seen from Table 5 that minimum release rates occurred when the cloud point was ~37°C. At this point the pore tortuosity within the matrix structure should also be at a maximum. It is unlikely to be an increase in viscosity that retards release rates since Ford *et al.* [1] showed that viscosity has little effect on release rates. Any reduction in hydration, such as that by increasing the concentration of solute in the dissolution media or increasing the temperature of the dissolution media, will start to prevent gelation and therefore the tablet will cease to act as a sustained release matrix.

The data produced here explains the results of Fassihi and Mundy [12] who explained the retardation of theophylline release into phosphate buffers in terms of a possible interaction between the phosphate and theophylline molecules. While this

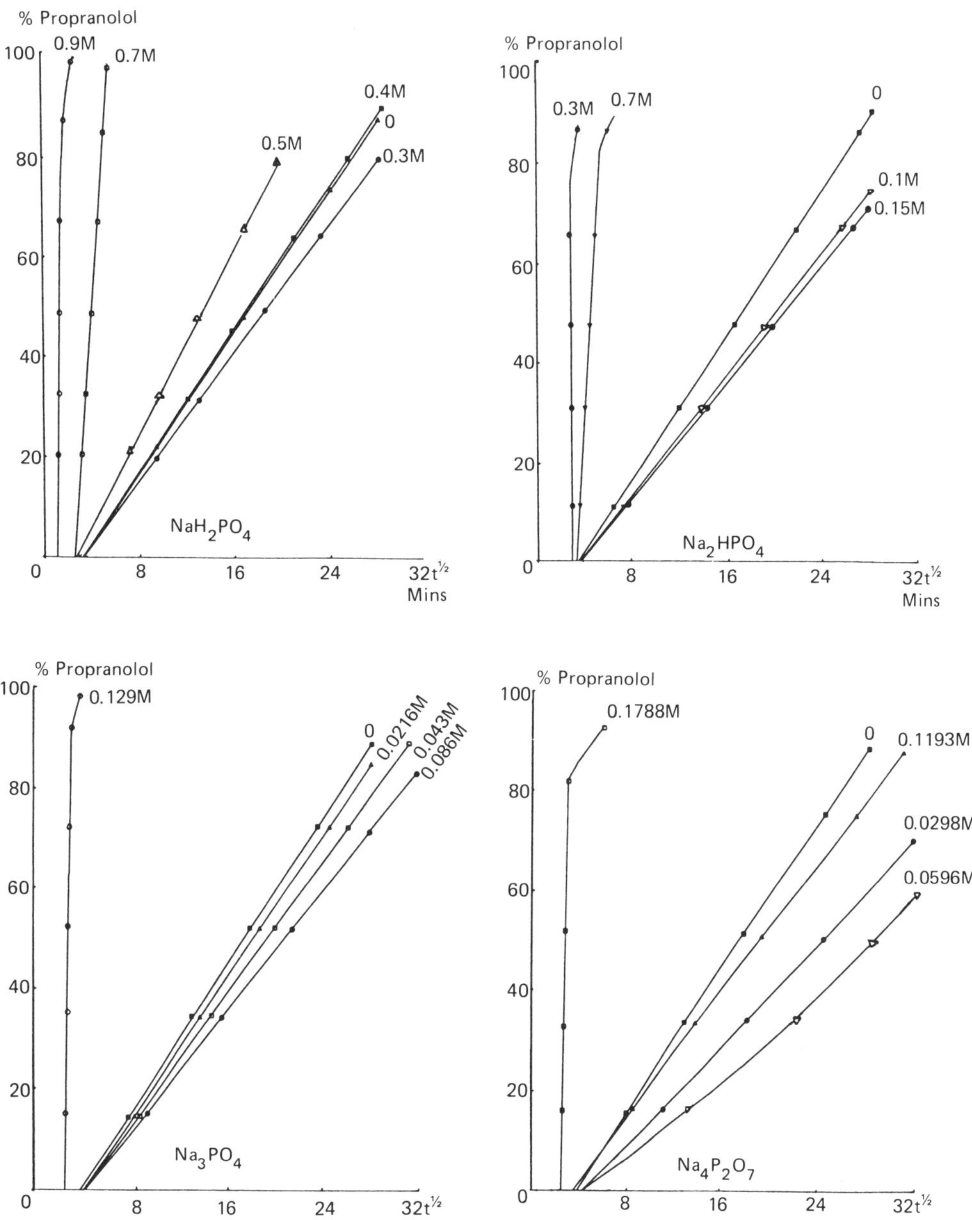

Fig. 2 — Dissolution profiles of propanolol hydrochloride from HPMC K15M matrices into media, buffered to pH 6.0 containing various solutes.

cannot be discounted, in view of the results reported it would seem unlikely that retardation was achieved by ionic strength effects since high levels of sodium chloride retarded drug release. Table 5 shows the relationship between the dissolution rates

Table 5 — The effect of solute and ionic strength in the dissolution rate of propranolol hydrochloride from HPMC K15M matrix tablets

Dissolution media (M)	Dissolution rate (% $min^{-\frac{1}{2}}$)	Ionic strength	Cloud point (°C)
Distilled water	3.999	—	68.2
NaH_2PO_4	4.115	0.1	58.8
	3.784	0.2	52.1
	3.578	0.3	46.0
	6.013	0.5	36.0
	Burst release	0.7	28.2
Na_2HPO_4	3.376	0.3	50.2
	3.200	0.36	47.3
	3.098	0.45	43.2
	3.092	0.6	37.1
	Burst release	0.9	27.4
Na_3PO_4	4.052	0.13	63.7
	3.623	0.258	56.8
	3.156	0.516	45.1
	Burst release	0.774	35.9
	3.155	1.193	57.8
$Na_4P_2O_7$	2.756	0.298	48.6
	2.381	0.596	34.3
	Burst release	1.788	24.3
NaCl	2.476	0.500	54.0

of propanolol hydrochloride from HPMC matrix tablets and the ionic strengths of the dissolution media. for the di-, tri- and tetravalent phosphate salts an ionic strength of approximately 0.6 produces minimum release rates from the tablets. The univalent phosphate salt produces a minimum release rate at an ionic strength of approximately 0.3. By examination of Table 5 it can be deduced that for burst release integrity need not be lost completely, e.g. using sodium dihydrogen orthophosphate as a medium an ionic strength of 0.7 is enough to produce burst release. However, the integrity is still maintained in disintegration studies for 53 min. This emphasizes the importance of the initial gelling of the HPMC to protect tablet integrity. When examining the dissolution rate of drugs from HPMC matrices it would seem that electrolytes added to the dissolution medium, even in small amounts, will modify the dissolution rate. It could well be that when studying the release at different pH values the changes in rates seen are not entirely due to changes in pH but are also due to the buffers used to produce that pH. Until further investigations are carried out and in order to avoid solute–HPMC interactions, it is suggested that only water should be used as the dissolution medium for fundamental studies into drug release. However, physiological conditions need to be considered further.

REFERENCES

[1] J. L. Ford, M. H. Rubinstein and J. E. Hogan, *Int. J. Pharm.*, **24**, 327 (1985).
[2] J. L. Ford, M. H. Rubinstein and J. E. Hogan, *Int. J. Pharm.*, **24**, 339 (1985).
[3] J. L. Ford, M. H. Rubinstein, F. McCaul, J. E. Hogan and P. J. Edgar, *Intg. Pharm.*, **40**, 223 (1987).
[4] N. Sarkar, *J. Appl. Polym. Sci.*, **24**, 1073, (1979).
[5] P. G. Fagan, P. J. Harrison and N. Shankland, *J. Pharm. Pharmacol.* (1989), in press.
[6] Alderman (1984).
[7] J. L. Ford, M. H. Rubinstein, A. Changela and J. A. Hogan, *J. Pharm. Pharmacol.*, **37**, 115P (1985).
[8] E. Touitou and M. Donbrow, *Int. J. Pharm.*, **11**, 131 (1982).
[9] A. T. Florence and R. T. Parfitt, *J. Pharm. Pharmacol.*, **22**, 121S (1970).
[10] G. Levy and T. W. Schwarz, *J. Am. Pharm. Assoc. Sci. Edn.*, **47**, 44 (1958).
[11] I. R. Katz and F. W. Muschter, *Biochem. Z.*, **257**, 385 (1933).
[12] A. R. Fasshi and D. L. Mundy, *J. Pharm. Pharmacol.*, **41**, 369 (1989).

3

Factors affecting the formulation of sustained release potassium chloride tablets

S. Şenel, Y. Çapan† and **A. A. Hncal**
Hacettepe University, Faculty of Pharmacy, Pharmaceutical Technology Department, 06100 Ankara, Turkey

SUMMARY

Compressed polymer matrices are widely used in sustained release. They are readily manufactured and make use of simple technology. However, they are among the most difficult to model and none can be relied on to produce true time-independent release. Despite these difficulties, many attempts have been made to improve and understand better the release kinetics.

In this study, the influence of several formulation factors on the release kinetics of potassium chloride from directly compressed matrices is investigated. Formulations containing hydrophilic (methylcellulose, carbomer), plastic (polyvinyl chloride) and wax (glycerol palmitostearate) matrix materials at concentrations of 10%, 15% and 20%, and insoluble excipients, were prepared and tested using the USP XXI–NF XVI rotating paddle method.

Hardness had no marked effect on release characteristics except for wax matrices. With hydrophilic matrices, for methylcellulose, increased matrix material concentration did not affect the release profile, but for carbomer, as the concentration increased, a significant decrease in released amount was obtained.

Goodness-of-fit analysis applied to release data showed that the release mechanism was described by the Higuchi diffusion-controlled model. Confirmation of the diffusion process is provided by the logarithmic form of an empirical equation ($M_t/M_\infty = kt^n$) given by Peppas. Positive deviations from the Higuchi equation might be due to air entrapped in the matrix and for hydrophilic matrices due to the erosion of the gel layer. Analysis of *in vitro* release indicated that the most suitable matrices were methylcellulose and glycerol palmitostearate.

† Author to whom correspondence should be addressed.

INTRODUCTION

Sustained release preparations of potassium chloride have been widely used to overcome the gastrointestinal side effects following medication with enteric coated tablets. Such formulation techniques delay the rate of absorption and produce a slow release of potassium chloride during the passage through the gastrointestinal tract [1,2].

Compressed polymeric matrices provide a convenient method for achieving sustained release of highly water-soluble drugs [3–5]. Release profiles are usually analysed by equations derived by T. Higuchi [6] and W. I. Higuchi [7].

MATERIALS AND METHODS

Materials

The following materials were used: potassium chloride (E. Merck, Darmstadt, FRG), polyvinyl chloride (Pevikon® PE 737P, Kemanord, Sweden), carbomer (Carbopol® 934 P, Goodrich, Zaventem, Belgium), glycerol palmitostearate (Precirol® ATO 5, Gattefosse, France), methylcellulose (Metolose® SM 4000, Shinetsu Chemical, Japan), dibasic calcium phosphate dihydrate (Emcompress® E. Mendell Co. Inc., New York, USA). magnesium stearate (E. Merck GmbH, FRG).

Methods

Preparation of tablets

Polyvinyl chloride, carbomer, methylcellulose and glycerol palmitostearate were used as matrix materials in this investigation. The powders were mixed and directly compressed with 1% of magnesium stearate incorporated as a lubricant prior to compression. Tablets were compressed on a single-punch tablet machine (Korsch EK/0) using a flat punch of 12 mm diameter at two different tablet hardnesses (3.5–4.0 kPa and 7.5–8 kPa). A Heberlein hardness tester was used. Sustained release matrix tablets were formulated to contain 600 mg (60% potassium chloride) and 10%, 15% or 20% matrix material of tablet weight. In order to obtain constant tablet weight, different percentages of dibasic calcium phosphate dihydrate as a filler were added.

In vitro release of potassium from tablets

Dissolution was carried out with the paddle method according to USP XXI, using a Prolabo dissolution tester. The dissolution medium was 1000 ml of distilled water at 37±0.5°C and 50 rev min^{-1}. At appropriate time intervals, 5 ml of sample was withdrawn and an equal volume of medium was added to maintain a constant volume. Sample were filtered, diluted with lithium carbonate solution as an internal standard, and analysed using a Dr Lange MD 70 flame photometer. Each dissolution profile is the average of six separate tablets.

RESULTS AND DISCUSSSION

Effect of polymer concentration

The results of the release experiments are summarized in Fig. 1 and Fig. 2, which represent the percentage released as a function of time. As expected, the drug was

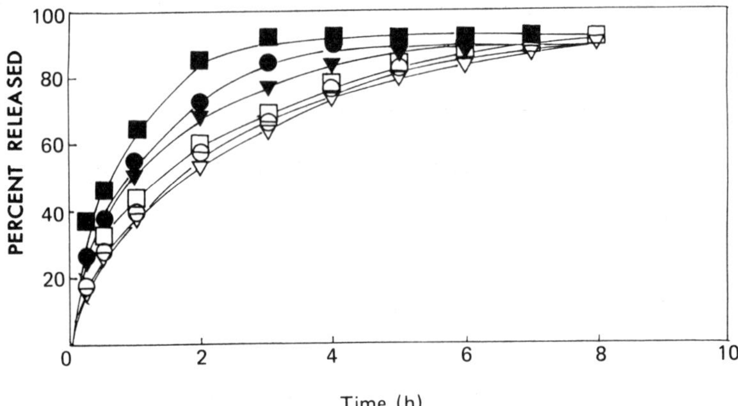

Fig. 1 — Potassium chloride release profiles from sustained release matrix tablets (hardness, 7.5–8 kp): 10% (■), 15% (●), 20% (▼) carbomer; 10% (□), 15% (○), 20% (▽) methylcellulose.

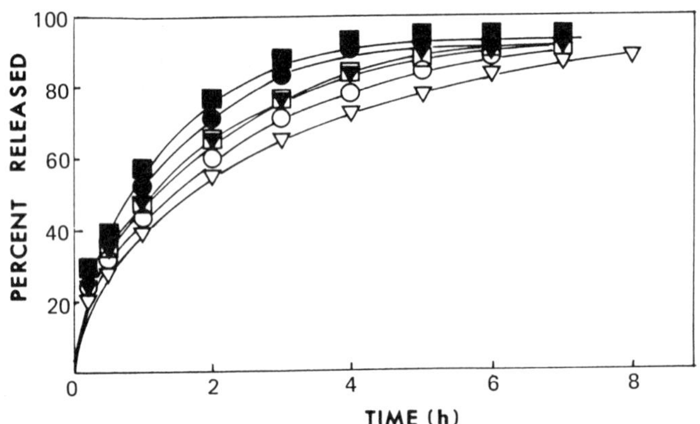

Fig. 2 — Potassium chloride release profiles from sustained release matrix tablets (hardness, 7.5–8 kp): 10% (■), 15% (●), 20% (▼) polyvinyl chloride; 10% (□), 15% (○), 20% (▽) glycerol palmitostearate.

released from tablets more slowly with an increase in polymer content. When 10%, 15% and 20% of carbomer were incorporated into the formulations (Fig. 1), the amount of potassium chloride decreased from 93% to 84–7% and 77.3% respectively at the end of 3 h. Glycerol palmitostearate showed similar results for the concentrations of 10%, 15% and 20%, i.e. the amount released was decreased, in 3 h, from 75.7% to 71.4% and 64.9% respectively (Fig. 2). Similar results were also obtained for polyvinyl chloride and methylcellulose. Carbomer and polyvinyl chloride matrix tablets show an initial rapid release of potassium chloride. While 52% and 48% of potassium chloride were released from 20% carbomer and polyvinyl chloride formulations, in 1 h, only 38% and 39% of potassium chloride were released from formulations containing 20% methylcellulose and glycerol palmitostearate respectively.

In order to investigate the mechanism of release, the following semi-empirical equation was used [8].

$$\frac{M_t}{M_\infty} = kt^n \tag{1}$$

where M_t/M_∞ is the fraction of drug released up to time t, k is a constant incorporating structural and geometric characteristics of the tablet, and n is the diffusional exponent indicative of the mechanism of release. The estimated parameters are given in Table 1.

Table 1 — Values of constant (k), release exponent (n) and correlation coefficient (r^2) following linear regression of dissolution data of formulations containing different polymers (hardness, 7.5–8 kp)

Matrix composition		Kinetic constant (k)	Release exponent (n) (mean±SD)	Coefficient of correlation (r^2)
Polyvinyl chloride	10%	0.519	0.447±0.063	0.980
	15%	0.557	0.473±0.042	0.980
	20%	0.480	0.453±0.024	0.990
Glycerol palmitostearate	10%	0.466	0.467±0.020	0.994
	15%	0.423	0.482±0.037	0.980
	20%	0.391	0.470±0.020	0.985
Methylcellulose	10%	0.445	0.402±0.034	0.970
	15%	0.369	0.583±0.037	0.984
	20%	0.374	0.517±0.032	0.982
Carbomer	10%	0.639	0.509±0.059	0.970
	15%	0.543	0.468±0.034	0.990
	20%	0.508	0.456±0.017	0.994

When equation (1) is applied during the early stages of release (fraction released <0.7) to geometries other than slabs (i.e. tablets), the value of the diffusional exponent, n, depends on the geometry of the system [8]. In the case of a cylinder,

Fickian diffusion is defined by n=0.45 and case II by n=0.89. The correct values of exponent n for different geometries are reported in Table 2.

Table 2 — Geometric dependence of diffusional exponent (n) of equation (1)

Diffusional exponent (n)			Transport mechanism
Slab	Cylinder	Sphere	
0.5	0.45	0.43	Fickian (case I)
>0.5	>0.45	>0.43	Anomalous
<1	<0.89	<0.85	
1	0.89	0.85	Case II

The anomalous behaviour for potassium chloride matrices with a value $n<0.5$ emphasizes the complex release of this drug. Peppas [8] did not interpret n values of <0.5 but stated that such occurrences were an indication of statistical analysis problems or were due to diffusion through a polymeric network where diffusion occurred partially through a swollen matrix and partly through water-filled pores. In this case, in order to investigate the mechanism of release, the percentage release v. time profile was evaluated for goodness of fit. The details of the use of this statistical technique are given by Bamba *et al.* [9] and Capan *et al.* [10]. They proposed the following mechansims which may be rate determining in the release of drug from a system: (a) the permeation of water; (b) the gelation rate; (c) the diffusion rate of drug in the gel; (d) the dissolution rate of the drug in penetrating water; (e) the Higuchi porous penetration [6]. If the release pattern of drug from the formula is dictated by process (a), (b) and (c), then it is first-order release and equation (2) should be applicable. If the release is represented by process (d), then a cube root relationship should hold (equation (3)), and if it is governed by porous penetration then the Higuchi square root law should apply equation (4).

$$\ln W = -k_f t + i \tag{2}$$

$$100^{1/3} - W^{1/3} = K_c t \tag{3}$$

$$100 - W = k_d t^{1/2} \tag{4}$$

where W is the percentage of drug undissolved at time t (h), k_f (h^{-1}) and i are the first-order dissolution rate constant and the intercept of the log–linear plot of the type in equation (2). k_c ($h^{1/3}$) is the cube root dissolution rate constant and k_d ($h^{-1/2}$)

is the Higuchi constant. To compare the data statistically, the dependent parameter must be in the same form (linear, logarithmic, etc.); therefore, the equations have been recast in the forms shown below, for comparison:

$$W = e^{i} e^{-k_{f} t} \tag{2a}$$

$$W = (100^{1/3} - k_{c} t)^{3} \tag{3a}$$

$$W = 100 - k_{d} t^{1/3} \tag{4a}$$

The goodness of fit was evaluated by the residuals and correlation coefficients are given in Table 3. For polyvinyl chloride, glycerol palmitostearate, carbomer and methylcellulose matrix tablets, equation (4) showed a significantly better fit than equations (2) and (3) by the F test.

Since carbomer is an hydrophilic matrix, it is expected that the release rate be governed by the gelation rate ($\ln W = -k_{f}t + i$). However, the best fit was obtained with the square root equation and the release rate constants determined from the slopes of the linear fit for carbomer matrix tablets are given in Table 4. Similar results were also obtained by Lapidus and Lordi [11], who applied the equations derived by Higuchi [6], and Desai *et al.* [12,13] for drug release from an insoluble matrix to a compressed hydrophilic matrix. Water penetration is visualized as hydrating the polymer and dissolving potassium chloride which then diffuses out through the swollen matrix. A decrease in the amount of carbomer causes a decrease in the embedding capacity of the matrix tablets (Table 4).

For methylcellulose, increased matrix material concentration did not affect the release profile (Table 4). The sustained action can be directly attributed to the formation of a hydration layer by this polymer. This hydration layer, however, did not resist attrition and remain intact. Consequently, attrition becomes more important than diffusion; the hydrated layer dissolves away almost as rapidly as it is formed. On the contrary, the dibasic calcium phosphate dihydrate did not diffuse outward, but rather became entrapped within the matrix and effected an increase in release of drug because its presence necessarily decreased the polymer concentration.

As the concentration of polyvinyl chloride and glycerol palmitostearate was increased between 15% and 20%, a non-significant decrease in released amount was obtained, while a slight difference in the amount released was observed beween 10% and 15% of polymer concentration (Table 4). Deviations from the Higuchi equation were observed (Table 3). These positive deviations might be due to the air entrapped in the matrix. Similar results were also obtained with polyvinyl chloride by Desai *et al.* [14] and Korsmeyer *et al.* [15].

Effect of tablet hardness

The effect of hardness on the release characteristics of potassium chloride is shown in Figs 3 and 4. The release rate constants for 15% polyvinyl chloride matrix tablets of

Table 3 — Comparison of fits using least-squares equations (hardness, 7.5–8 kp)

Formulation		First order (equation (2a))		Square root (equation (4a))		Cube root (equation (3a))	
Matrix material	Amount (%)	r^2	$\frac{\Sigma(\text{residuals})^2}{n-2}$	r^2	$\frac{\Sigma(\text{residuals})^2}{n-2}$	r^2	$\frac{\Sigma(\text{residuals})^2}{n-2}$
Polyvinyl chloride	10	0.802	197.08	0.969	37.88	0.835	144.00
	15	0.665	361.69	0.890	83.51	0.693	279.06
	20	0.806	188.34	0.976	17.59	0.841	133.49
Glycerol palmitostearate	10	0.740	269.48	0.952	36.16	0.777	206.19
	15	0.757	240.96	0.964	26.31	0.798	168.51
	20	0.786	195.89	0.981	13.02	0.829	130.86
Methylcellulose	10	0.804	166.80	0.980	13.26	0.839	118.16
	15	0.738	309.16	0.968	26.21	0.789	198.05
	20	0.773	229.83	0.982	13.35	0.823	147.34
Carbomer	10	0.836	177.08	0.976	21.11	0.865	131.58
	15	0.837	157.99	0.982	13.96	0.868	113.22
	20	0.766	190.66	0.960	26.89	0.802	142.46

Table 4 — Release rate constants ($h^{1/2}$) of tablets

Formulation		4 kp hardness: release rate constant ($h^{-1/2}$) (mean±SD (CV))	8 kp hardness: release rate constant ($h^{-1/2}$) (mean±SD (CV))
Matrix material	Amount (%)		
Polyvinyl chloride	10	38.91±1.29 (3.3%)	36.03±2.78 (7.7%)
	15	32.40±0.93 (2.9%)	33.99±4.22 (12.4%)
	20	32.77±1.05 (3.2%)	33.71±2.09 (6.2%)
Glycerol palmitostearate	10	34.29±1.53 (4.5%)	34.44±1.28 (3.7%)
	15	28.82±1.01 (3.5%)	31.29±1.86 (5.9%)
	20	30.14±1.01 (3.4%)	30.00±0.96 (3.2%)
Methylcellulose	10	34.59±1.88 (5.4%)	29.55±1.02 (3.5%)
	15	31.02±0.83 (2.7%)	33.37±1.52 (4.5%)
	20	30.77±1.21 (3.9%)	31.37±0.92 (2.9%)
Carbomer	10	47.03±1.27 (2.7%)	50.96±1.97 (3.9%)
	15	41.88±1.04 (2.5%)	41.90±0.89 (2.1%)
	20	32.20±0.47 (1.5%)	32.66±0.46 (1.4%)

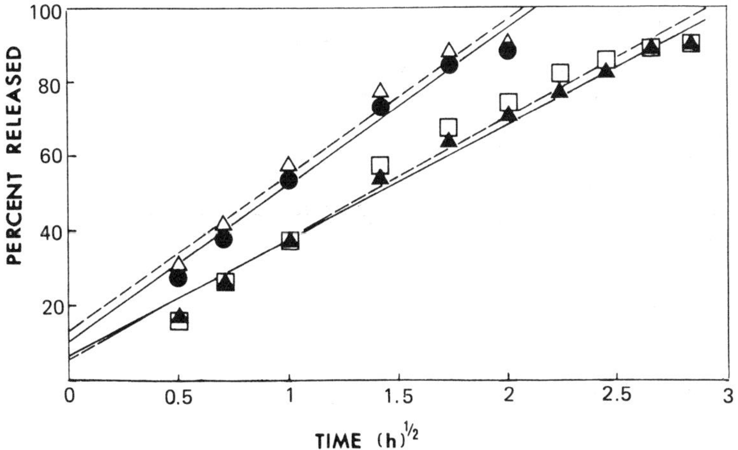

Fig. 3 — A plot of the percentage released against the square root of time showing the effect of tablet hardness (matrix material concentration, 15%): carbomer, △, 3.5–4 kp; ●, 7.5–8 kp; methylcellulose, ▲, 3.5–4 kp; □, 7.5–8 kp.

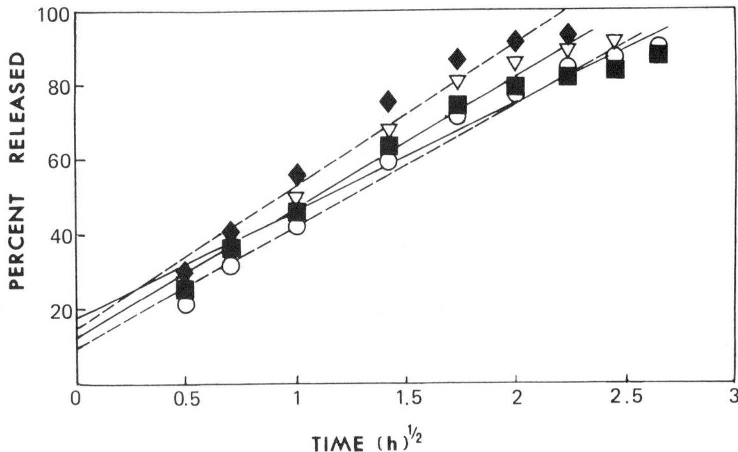

Fig. 4 — A plot of the percentage released against the square root of time showing the effect of tablet hardness (matrix material concentration, 15%): polyvinyl chloride, ◆, 3.5–4 kp; ▽, 7.5–8 kp; glycerol palmitostearate, ■, 3.5–4 kp, ○, 7.5–8 kp.

4 kp and 8 kp hardness were 32.40±0.93 and 33.99±4.22 respectively. No significant differences in the release rate constants were observed ($p>0.05$).

The porosity and density of the tablets were not determined. From a theoretical standpoint, hardness measurements quantitatively reflect differences in density and porosity of the tablets. These could possibly influence the rate of tablet dissolution by afffecting the initial rate of penetration of dissolution fluid at the tablet surface. This, in turn, would affect the rate of formation of the gel barrier at the periphery for the carbomer and methylcellulose matrix tablets. The results thus indicate that one can expect little or no change in release pattern as a result of alteration in tablet density and porosity of the system. If, however, changes occur, they will probably appear during the initial phase of the dissolution period, and the shape of the release profile will not be markedly altered. The effect of hardness on the release profiles of tablets prepared by using polyvinyl chloride and glycerol palmitostearate was also given by other investigators [12–15], and was in accordance with our results.

This study indicates that drug release from these formulations is by a matrix-diffusion-controlled process. The release rate constant shows an inverse relationship with the concentration of carbomer only. For all the formulations, release rate constants were independent of tablet hardness.

REFERENCES

[1] J. A. Rider, R. J. Manner and J. I. Swader, *J. Am. Med. Assoc.*, **231**, 836 (1975).
[2] D. Ben-Ishay and K. Engelman, *Clin. Pharmacol. Ther.*, **14**, 250 (1973).
[3] H. E. Huber, L. B. Dale and G. L. Christenson, *J. Pharm. Sci.*, **55**, 974 (1966).

[4] H. E. Huber and G. L. Christenson, *J. Pharm. Sci.*, **57**, 164 (1968).
[5] Y. Çapan, *Drug Dev. Ind. Pharm.*, **15**, 927 (1989).
[6] T. Higuchi, *J. Pharm. Sci.*, **52**, 1145 (1963).
[7] W. I. Higuchi, *J. Pharm. Sci.*, **51**, 802 (1962).
[8] N. A. Peppas, *Pharm. Acta. Helv.*, **60**, 110 (1985).
[9] M. Bamba, F. Puisieux, J. P. Marty and J. T. Carstensen, *Int. J. Pharm.*, **2**, 307 (1979).
[10] Y. Çapan, S. Şenel, S. Çals, S. Takka and A. A. Hncal, *Pharm. Ind.*, **51**, 443 (1989).
[11] H. Lapidus and N. G. Lordi, *J. Pharm. Sci.*, **57**, 1292 (1968).
[12] S. J. Desai, P. Singh, A. P. Simonelli and W. I. Higuchi, *J. Pharm. Sci.*, **54**, 1459 (1965).
[13] S. J. Desai, P. Singh, A. P. Simonelli and W. I. Higuchi, *J. Pharm. Sci.*, **55**, 1224 (1966).
[14] S. J. Desai, P. Singh, A. P. Simonelli and W. I. Higuchi, *J. Pharm. Sci.*, **55**, 1235 (1966).
[15] R. W. Korsmeyer, R. Gurny, E. Doelker, P. Buri and N. A. Peppas, *J. Pharm. Sci.*, **72**, 1189 (1983).

4

Statistical optimization of a controlled release formulation obtained by a double-compression process: Application of a Hadamard matrix and a factorial design

A. Peña Romero
Laboratoire de Pharmacie Galénique et Industrielle, UFR de Pharmacie de Grenoble, Avenue de Verdun, 38243 Meylan, France
J. B. Costa and **I. Castel-Maroteaux**
Searle Recherche et Développement, Sophia Antipolis, 06560 Valbonne, France
and
D. Chulia
Laboratoire de Pharmacie Galénique et Industrielle, UFR de Pharmacie de Grenoble, Avenue de Verdun, 38243 Meylan, France

SUMMARY

A formulation containing an anti-inflammatory agent (diclofenac sodium), two inert matrices (ethylcellulose and polyvinyl chloride), a lubricant (magnesium stearate) and talc was optimized and prepared by a double compression process.

In the first stage, preliminary trials were performed in order to study the effect of lubricant added before and after precompression.

A Hadamard matrix H(8) was applied to estimate the main effects of four parameters: applied force at the upper punch (UPF) during precompression, UPF during the final compression, particle size range after milling and the concentration of ethylcellulose added before the final compression.

According to the Hadamard matrix, a 2^2 factorial design was built. The complete linear models were fitted by regression for each response, reflecting the compression behaviour and dissolution kinetics.

Validation was carried out using the area under the dissolution curve, this being the major response to be optimized. The dissolution curves fitted the Weibull distribution.

INTRODUCTION

Dry granulation is a process which consists of granulating a powder by compression, avoiding the wetting and drying steps. The advantages and drawbacks of this process were described by Sheth *et al.* [1]. The two methods used for dry granulation are compaction and double compression [2,3].

Two polymers were incorporated in the inert matrix system: ethylcellulose and polyvinyl chloride. The processes used to prepare tablets containing such polymers often include direct compression [4–6], wet granulation [7,8], coating [9–11] and, rarely, dry granulation [12].

In previous work, the formula used were optimized by direct compression [13]. The area under the dissolution curve was optimized and validated by a composite design. However, the formulation gave poor powder flow as well as variability in the dissolution parameters. Thus the double compression process was investigated in order to change the powder into solid aggregates and therefore to enhance homogeneity, density and powder flow; in addition it was expected that this process would reduce the variability between tablets.

Statistical optimization was conducted in three steps:

(1) A Hadamard matrix H(8) was first applied to study the main effects of four parameters.
(2) A 2^2 factorial design was built to obtain a complete linear model including only two parameters.
(3) Validation of the mathematical model and then the optimum formulation were then made.

MATERIALS

The formula contained the drug, two inert matrices and two lubricants:

Diclofenac sodium (Secifarma) 25.0%
Ethylcellulose N-7 (Hercules) 26.1%
PVC (Pevikon PE 737 P) (SEPPIC) 45.9%
Magnesium stearate (Prophac) 1.0%
Talc USP (Prophac) 2.0%

METHODS

The manufacturing process

When using dry granulation, it is highly desirable to add a binder to the mixture in order to ensure an acceptable cohesion between particles. Therefore, in this present study, ethylcellulose was incorporated in two parts: before precompression as a binder, and before the final compression as an independent variable in the experimental design.

The manufacturing process described below was followed:

(1) Mixing for 5 min in a Turbula WAB (T2C, Willy A. Bachofen AG).
(2) Precompression using a Frogerais 0A single-punch instrumented press (Ets. Ed. Frogerais), equipped with flat punches 11.28 mm in diameter (surface area, 1 cm^2). The speed of the machine was adjusted to one tablet s^{-1}.
(3) Milling was carried out in an Erweka oscillating granulator equipped with 3.15 mm perforations for premilling and 0.8 mm perforations for the final milling.
(4) Grinding and separation of the particle size ranges in a Russell vibratory machine (Russell Finex, London and New York).
(5) Lubrication for 3 min.
(6) Final compression on the same instrumented tablet machine to obtain a 400 mg tablet.

TESTS PERFORMED

Powder test

Powder flow rate was determined using a glass funnel. The volume before and after tapping ($\Delta V = V_{10} - V_{500}$) was measured with an Eberhard Bauer (J. Engelsmann AG) tapping volume meter [14–16].

Physics of compression

In sampling ten tablets, the following parameters were studied: the lubrication index (R), the ejection force (F_e), the residual force (F_r) and the cohesion index (CI=ratio of the pressure applied to the upper punch and the tensile strength) proposed by Guyot [17].

In one of the ten tablets, the mechanical work was calculated using the parameter of the total energy liberated during the compression (E_t).

In sampling 120 tablets, the friability, the variability of the tablet weight and the variability of the upper punch force were determined.

Tablet tests

Friability was determined with 20 tablet samples in a friability tester (Erweka TA3R; 15 min, 25 rev min^{-1}).

The weight variation was evaluated for 20 tablets on an electronic balance (Mettler AK 260; Sofranie).

Tablet hardness was measured on 10 tablets using a Schleuniger hardness tester (Soteco).

Dissolution studies

Six tablets were subjected to dissolution using the USP dissolution apparatus (Vanderkamp 600, Van-Kel Ind., NJ, USA) in 500 ml buffer pH 1.2 (the first hour) and 650 ml buffer pH 6.8 (1–14 h), maintained at 37°C and rotated with paddles at 50 rev min^{-1} (first hour) and 130 rev min^{-1} (1–14 h). The dissolution apparatus was connected to a UV–visible spectrophotometer (Uvikon 810, Roxche Bioéléctronique Kontron, Marseille) and a computer (VAX 780; Digital). The absorbance of the dissolution medium at 275 nm was recorded automatically at intervals (1, 2, 4, 5, 8,

10, 12 and 14 h). The percentage of the drug released was calculated and the corresponding release profiles were obtained.

PRELIMINARY TRIALS

The objective of the preliminary trials was to define the best way to incoporate the lubricants, i.e. before or after the precompression operation. Three experiments were carried out.

(1) *Experiment A.* Talc was added before precompression and magnesium stearate before the final compression.
(2) *Experiment B.* 50% of each lubricant was incorporated before and after precompression.
(3) *Experiment C.* Magnesium stearate was mixed before precompression and talc before the final compression.

In these three experiments, 50% of the ethylcellulose was added before precompression and the other 50% before the final compression.

Precompression was conducted at 10 kN (UPF) and a 10 mm depth of the die. After milling and grinding, the 100–800 μm particle size range was collected and lubricated. For final compression, the powder was compresseed at 10 kN.

Results and discussion

Results obtained from the preliminary trials described above are shown in Table 1. The mean values of three trials performed for validation of the optimized formulation by direct compression [13] are given for comparison. The release profiles are illustrated in Fig. 1.

As expected, the flow rate, ΔV, R, F_e, F_r, E_t, UPF variation and weight variation were better than for direct compression. CI and friability were affected owing to the poor crushing strength (hardness) of the tablets obtained after the final compression.

Double compression largely decreases the coefficients of variation of the percentage dissolved at 8 h and AUC.

Adding lubricants before or after precompression reveals an effect on the different studied properties. Experiments A and B give better values than experiment C. In addition, the parameters R, F_e, F_r and CI are affected when talc is added alone before the final compression.

In conclusion, the incorporation of 50% magnesium stearate and talc before precompression and the other 50% before the final compression improves the compression behaviour. At the same time, it decreases the coefficients of variation of UPF the weight of the tablet and dissolution parameters. From these results, the process from experiment B was chosen for the experimental designs.

APPLICATION OF A HADAMARD MATRIX H(8)

Experimental design

The theory and application of a Hadamard matrix were discussed by Ozil and Rochat [18]. This design is an optimum strategy leading to good accuracy in the main effects

Table 1 — Precompression and final compression lubrication

Parameter		Experiment A	Experiment B	Experiment C	Direct compression
Powder flow rate (g/sec)		16.7	16.7	9.0	0.0
ΔV (ml)		21.0	18.0	17.0	52.0
R	PC	0.73	0.76	0.84	0.82
	FC	0.88	0.87	0.79	
F_e (kN)	PC	0.50	0.32	0.16	0.21
	FC	0.17	0.18	0.33	
F_r (kN)	PC	0.56	0.34	0.13	0.17
	FC	0.05	0.06	0.23	
Cohesion	PC	84	84	78	71
index	FC	91	130	385	
E_t (N m)	PC	37.1	34.8	34.6	33.5
	FC	21.6	19.7	19.2	
UPF variation (CV, %)		2.5	1.9	2.2	4.0
Weight variation (CV, %)		1.1	0.4	0.8	1.8
Friability (%)		0.83	1.14	1.65	0.09
% dissolved at 8 h		63.7	88.4	109.8	56.5
(CV, %)		5.3	1.1	1.1	12.4
AUC (% h)		657	975	1226	667
(CV, %)		7.6	1.7	1.6	9.0

PC, precompression; FC, final compression.

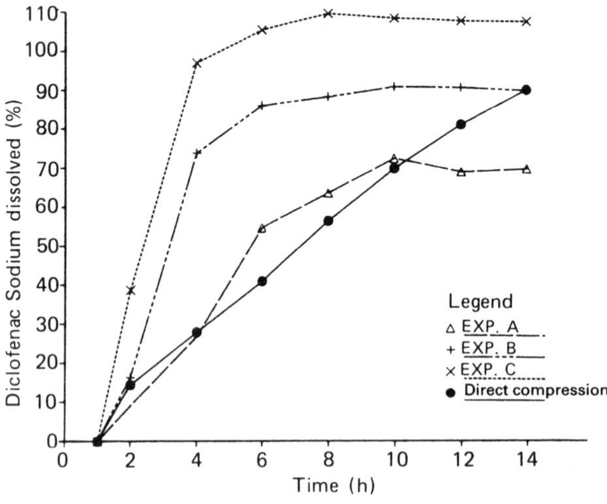

Fig. 1 — Release profiles of preliminary trials.

from a minimal number of experiments (N parameters+1=number which is a power of 2). With the coefficients (b_i) a linear model can be found for a given response Y:

$$Y = b_0 + b_1X_1 + b_2X_2 + b_3X_3 + \ldots + b_nX_n + \text{residue}$$

X_i is a reduced variable associated with each parameter P_i:

$$X_i = [2(P_i - P_{\text{mean}})/(P_{\text{maxima}} - P_{\text{minima}})]$$

Four independent variables were chosen for optimizing flow, compression behaviour and dissolution kinetics. Table 2 lists these four variables and their experimental ranges (levels). In order to decrease friability and CI, the percentage of ethylcellulose before the final compression was decreased.

Table 3 shows the responses to be optimized, among which AUC was considered the most important. A constant release between 1 and 12 h (passing through 60% dissolved at 8 h) and a complete dissolution after 14 h were chosen for an optimum profile (AUC=713% h).

Table 2 — Independent variable levels

P_i	Values for the following X_i levels	−1	+1
P_1:	UPF during precompression (kN)	8	12
P_2:	particle size range (μm)	100–400	400–800
P_3:	UPF at the final compression (kN)	8	12
P_4:	ethylcellulose before the final compression (%)	20	30

As four parameters were studied, three dummy variables X_5, X_6 and X_7 were included to build a Hadamard matrix H(8) composed of seven parameters:

Table 3 — Optimized responses

Y_i	Responses	Optimal values
Y_1	$\Delta V = V_{10} - V_{500}$ (ml)	<20
Y_2	Cohesion index	<100
Y_3	Weight variation (CV, %)	<1
Y_4	Friability of tablets (%)	<1
Y_5	Drug dissolved at 8 h (%)	~60
Y_6	AUC (% h)	~713
Y_7	Coefficient of variation of Y_5 (%)	<5
Y_8	Coefficient of variation of Y_6 (%)	<5

$$
\begin{array}{c|cccccccc}
X_i & & 1 & 2 & 3 & 4 & 5 & 6 & 7 \\
 & 1 & -1 & 1 & 1 & 1 & 1 & 1 & 1 \\
 & 1 & -1 & 1 & -1 & 1 & -1 & 1 & -1 \\
 & 1 & 1 & -1 & -1 & 1 & 1 & -1 & -1 \\
\mathbf{H}(8)= & 1 & -1 & -1 & 1 & 1 & -1 & -1 & 1 \\
 & 1 & 1 & 1 & 1 & -1 & -1 & -1 & -1 \\
 & 1 & -1 & 1 & -1 & -1 & 1 & -1 & 1 \\
 & 1 & 1 & -1 & -1 & -1 & -1 & 1 & 1 \\
 & 1 & -1 & -1 & 1 & -1 & 1 & 1 & -1
\end{array}
$$

Columns 1–4 lead to the matrix of experiments. According to the original units (Table 2), eight trials were carried out (Table 4). To avoid systematic errors, the trials were performed in random order.

Table 4 — Experimental design

Experiment	$P1$ (kN)	$P2$ (μm)	$P8$ (kN)	$P4$ (%)
1	12	400–800	12	30
2	8	400–800	8	30
3	12	100–400	8	30
4	8	100–400	12	30
5	12	400–800	12	20
6	8	400–800	8	20
7	12	100–400	8	20
8	8	100–400	12	20

The analysis of variance (ANOVA) gives information on the significant effects. Data were analyzed using the general linear model (GLM) procedure from the Statistical Analysis System (SAS Institute, Cary, NC). A discussion and explanation of the statistics involved are given by Davies [19].

The responses Y_2, Y_5 and Y_6 were transformed into natural logarithms to homogenize the distribution of the residues. Then, the F test was used to determine the statistical significance of the effects. An effect was considered as significant when $F>4(4=F_{0.95}(1,60)$.

Results and discussion

Table 5 contains results for each dependent variable. The release profiles are illustrated in Fig. 2.

ANOVA shows that X_2 is the most significant variable. It explains the variability of the main responses (Table 6).

In addition, for Y_6, the principal response to be optimized, X_2, X_3 and X_4 are all significant. The ln Y_6 model estimated by regression is (error, $s=0.04$, DF=44; $R^2=0.91$, $p=0.05$)

$$\ln Y_6=6.93-0.11X_2-0.03X_3-0.03X_4$$

From the models, when X_2, X_3 and X_4 decrease, the dissolution parameters increase. This can be explained by the hydrophobic effect of the ethylcellulose (X_4). Furthermore, an increased effective drug surface area occurs when the particle size range and the UPF at the final compression are at minimal levels and an increase in dissolution rate occurs. The area under the dissolution curve is far above the optimum value (713% h). Another experimental design must be explored.

FACTORIAL DESIGN: SEARCHING FOR AN OPTIMUM

Design

In order to improve Y_6 and according to the linear model previously found for this response, it was decided to fix X_1 and X_2 at -1 (8 kN) and $+1$ (400–800 μm) levels respectively; then, a 2^2 factorial design was built with the two other significant parameters X_3 and X_4 at the upper levels.

Table 7 gives the experimental and physical units of this factorial design.

Results and discussion

As shown in Table 8, the AUC (Y_6) from experiment 12 is near the optimum value. Y_2, Y_3 and Y_4 were also improved while Y_7 and Y_8 were affected. The release profiles are presented in Fig. 3.

The complete linear models were determined by regression (Table 9). The R^2 values for ln Y_2, Y_4, ln Y_5 ln Y_6 and mainly for Y_3 are quite low, indicating that the linear model is inadequate for describing the situation for these variables and that a quadratic model could better fit the data. Nevertheless, Y_6 from experiment 12 is a good value, as well as the other responses in this trial and may produce the optimum.

Validity of the optimum formulation

Two trials were carried out using the same levels as experiment 12: $P_1=8$ kN, $P_2=400$–800 μm, $P_3=12$ kN and $P_4=35\%$ ethylcellulose. Table 10 gives the results of the three trials in this validation. The predicted responses from the linear models and the relative errors are presented. If Y_3, Y_4 and Y_8 present the worst case, the results on the main responses are suitable.

Linearization of the dissolution data

Drug release from controlled release matrix tablets has been described by many kinetic theories [20,21]. Fig. 4 illustrates the release profiles of the validated dissolution (experiments 12, 12b and 12c) and the release profiles obtained from fits to the Weibull, Higuchi and Hixson–Crowell models. Figs 5 and 6 show the curves after linear transformation.

Table 5 — Hadamard matrix **H**(8) results

Experiment	Y_1	Y_2	Y_3	Y_4	Y_5	Y_6	Y_7	Y_8
1	12	126	0.55	0.78	85.7	869	3.2	4.6
2	17	332	1.68	2.73	84.1	892	4.9	6.9
3	18	123	0.44	1.80	98.5	1159	0.7	2.6
4	20	132	1.71	0.91	94.2	1041	0.9	0.9
5	16	169	0.83	0.93	87.0	910	3.8	5.4
6	14	126	0.30	1.30	91.4	997	0.9	1.2
7	33	169	0.52	2.63	99.3	1197	1.2	0.7
8	26	84	0.50	0.75	100.0	1135	0.7	2.2

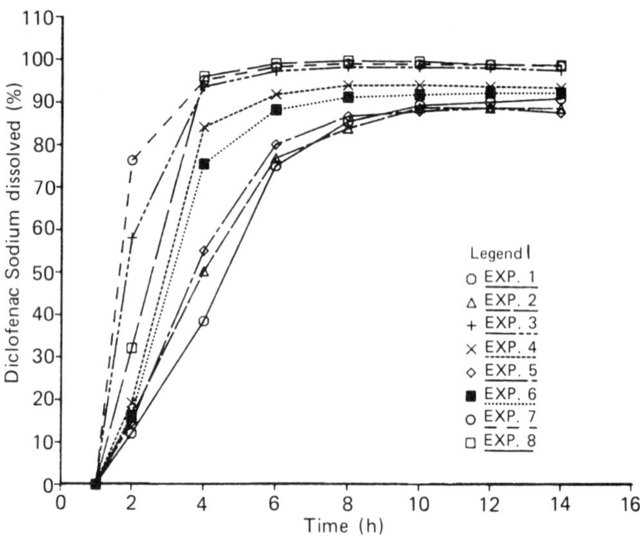

Fig. 2 — Release profiles from the study of main effects.

Table 11 contains the pertinent parameter estimates and the residual error for each release model. From these results and from Figs 4, 5 and 6 it can be concluded that the release of diclofenac sodium is fitted by the Weibull distribution. $\beta>1$ (β being the shape parameter) is characteristic for a slower initial rate (diclofenac sodium is insoluble at pH 1.2) followed by an acceleration to the final plateau (sigmoid). In the direct compression optimization, after 'infinite' time, the fraction released ($F-_{\infty}$) is estimated to be only 90% [13].

Table 6 — Results from the analysis of variance (F values)

Source of variation	Y_1	ln Y_2	Y_3	Y_4	ln Y_5	ln Y_6	Y_7	Y_8
X_1	0.0	0	1.2	0.1	0	1	0.1	0.1
X_2	6.6	25	0.0	0.0	194	347	4.6	3.3
X_3	0.3	23	0.1	7.2	4	37	0.0	0.1
X_4	2.2	9	1.7	0.1	24	37	0.5	0.7
s	5.24	0.31	0.61	0.67	0.03	0.04	1.54	2.27
DF	3	75	3	3	43	43	3	3

Table 7 — 2^2 factorial design

Experiment	Experimental units		Physical units	
	X_3	X_4	P_3 (kN)	P_4 (%)
9	1	1	18	40
10	−1	1	12	40
11	1	−1	18	35
12	−1	−1	12	35

Table 8 — Results from the 2^2 factorial design

Experiment	Y_1	Y_2	Y_3	Y_4	Y_5	Y_6	Y_7	Y_8
9	13	101	0.47	0.40	49.5	603	13.2	5.8
10	13	101	0.81	0.39	65.0	667	9.7	4.5
11	13	91	0.99	0.31	55.6	622	12.1	6.6
12	13	96	0.36	0.45	72.3	721	8.3	4.3

CONCLUSION

From a minimum number of experiments, the Hadamard matrix gives the possibility of estimating the mean effects of four parameters. Among them, the particle size range had the most important effect in the release of diclofenac sodium. By

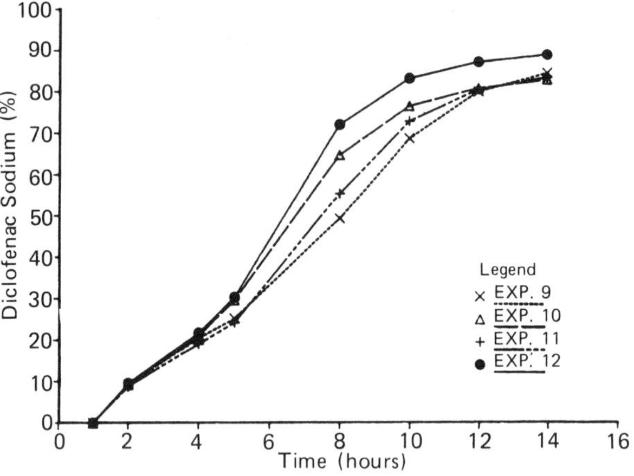

Fig. 3 — Release profiles from the factorial design.

Table 9 — Complete linear models

Coefficient	ln Y_2	Y_3	Y_4	ln Y_5	ln Y_6	Y_7	Y_8
b_0	4.57	0.66	0.39	4.09	6.48	10.83	5.30
b_3	−0.01	0.07	−0.03	−0.13	−0.06	1.83	0.90
b_4	0.04	−0.02	0.01	−0.06	−0.03	0.63	−0.15
b_3b_4	0.01	—	—	−0.0	0.01	—	—
Residual error							
s	0.054	0.485	0.075	0.108	0.053	0.150	0.500
DF	36	1	1	20	20	1	1
R^2	0.42	0.09	0.44	0.69	0.67	0.99	0.93

interpreting data, a factorial design including only two parameters was applied from which an optimum formulation was found.

As expected, when compared with the direct compression results [13], double compression considerably enhanced the flow of the powder and substantially decreased the variability between tablets. The drug release followed the Weibull distribution.

The inert matrix formulation provided by ethylcellulose and Pevikon (polyvinyl chloride) was an effective vehicle for controlled release drug delivery systems.

ACKNOWLEDGEMENTS

The authors express their gratitude to A. T. Luong, general manager of Searle, Sophia Antipolis, for his helpful comments.

Table 10 — Validity of the optimum formulation

Experiment	Y_2	Y_3	Y_4	Y_5	Y_6	Y_7	Y_8
12	96	0.36	0.45	72.3	721	8.3	4.3
12b	91	0.82	0.52	69.0	690	10.3	6.9
12c	88	0.56	0.57	68.5	691	6.2	3.5
Relative error							
Predicted response	95	0.61	0.41	72.2	721	8.4	4.6
Mean response	92	0.58	0.51	69.9	701	8.3	4.9
CV (%)	4.4	39.8	11.7	3.0	2.5	24.8	36.3
Residue	−3	−0.03	0.10	−2.3	−20	−0.1	0.3
Relative error —%)	3.3	5.2	19.6	3.3	2.9	1.2	6.1

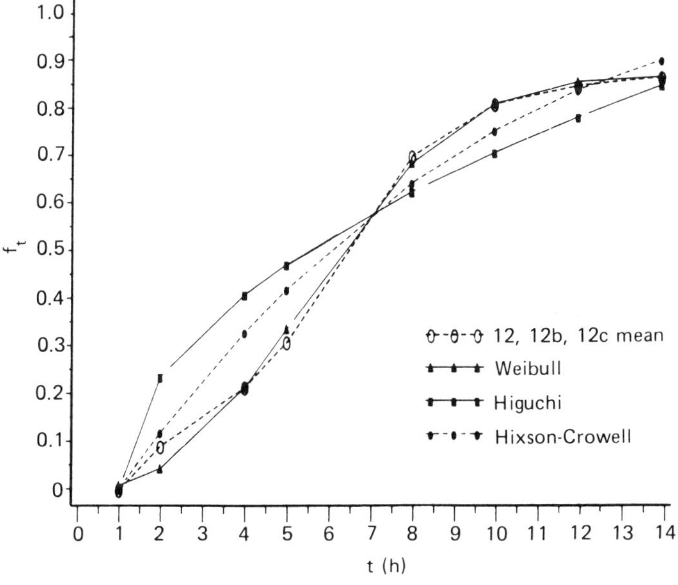

Fig. 4 — Mean data dissolution and theoretical release profiles.

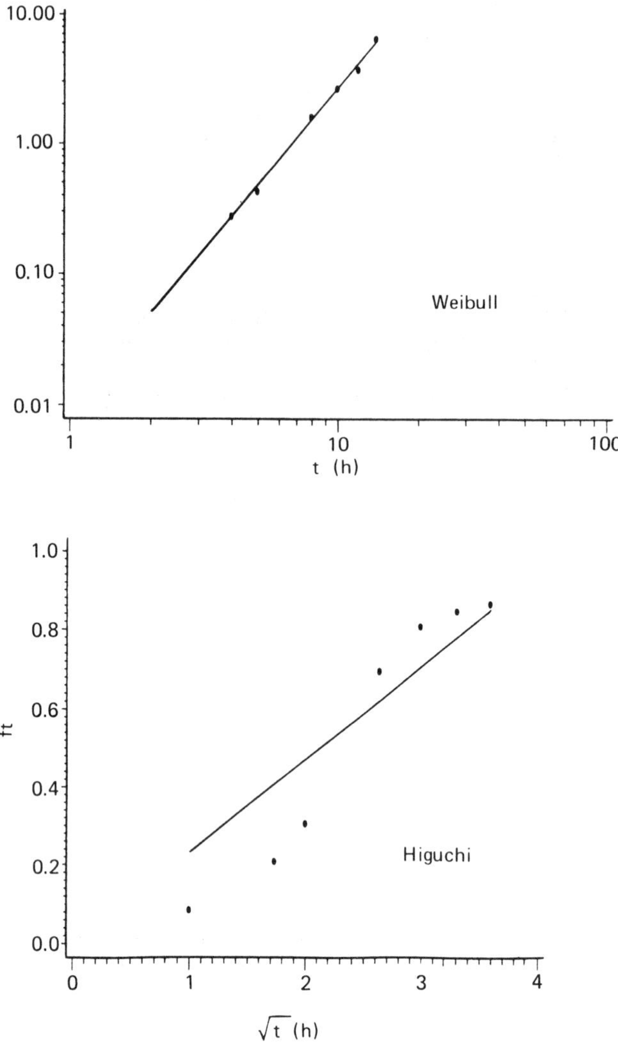

Fig. 5 — Linearization of the release profiles: Weibull and Higuchi models.

Angelina Peña Romero wishes to thank El Consejo Nacional de Ciencia y Tecnología, La Facultad de Estudios Superiores de la Universidad Nacional Autónoma de México, Le Comité d'Etudes sur la Formation d'Ingénieurs, Paris, and Searle, Sophia Antipolis, for their moral and financial support.

REFERENCES

[1] B. B. Sheth, F. J. Bandelin and R. F. Shangraw, in *Pharmaceutical Dosage Forms: Tablets,* Vol. 1, Dekker, New York, 1980, pp. 127–128, 173, 177.

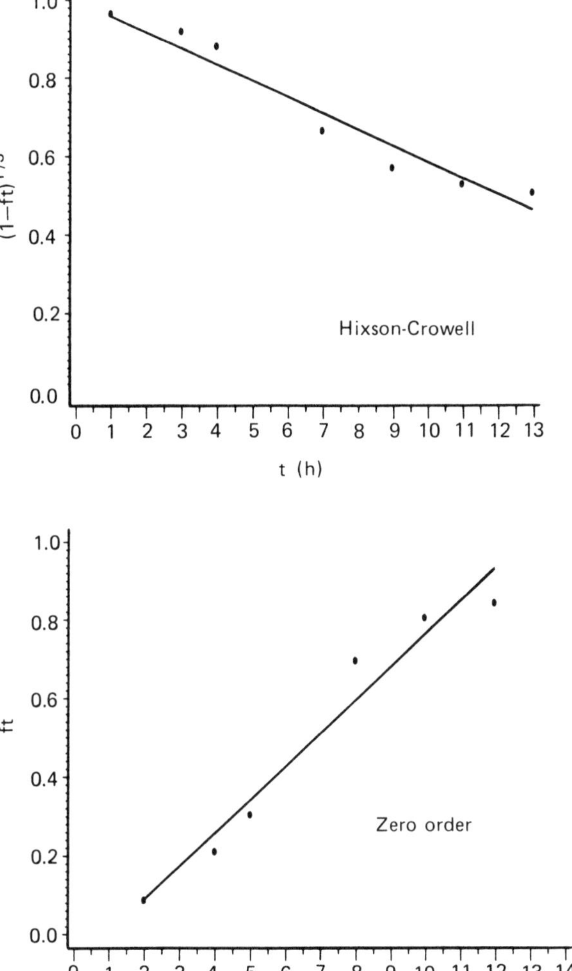

Fig. 6 — Linearization of the release profiles: Hixson–Crowell and zero-order models.

[2] A. Peña Romero, J. B. Costa and D. Chulia, *J. Pharm. Belg.*, to be submitted.
[3] A. Peña Romero, J. B. Costa, D. Chulia and A. T. Luong, *5th International Conf. on Pharmaceutical Technology, APGI, Paris, 1989.*
[4] M. H. Rutz-Coudray, J. Giust and P. Buri, *Pharm. Acta Helv.*, **54**, 363 (1979).
[5] A. R. Fassihi, *Int. J. Pharm.*, **37**, 119 (1987).
[6] C. Thomas, *Thesis,* University of Bourgogne, France, 1987.
[7] S. Chandrashekhar, S. B. Jayaswal and K. D. Gode, *Indian J. Hosp. Pharm.*, **14**, 72 (1977).
[8] M. L. Costa, H. Fessi and J. P. Marty, *Pharm. Acta Helv.*, **61**, 298 (1986).

Table 11 — Results from the fits to theoretical dissolution models

	Weibull	Higuchi	Hixson–Crowell	Zero-order ($f_t=a+K_0t$)
Parameter estimates	$F_\infty=0.87$ $t_0=0$ $t_d=6.70$ $\beta=2.46$	$K_H=0.235$	$K_{HC}=0.041$	$a=-0.081$ $K_0=0.084$
σ^2 estimate	0.0016	0.0163	0.0025	0.0051

σ^2 is estimated by the MS residual (sum of Squares)DF).

[9] F. W. Goodhart, M. R. Harris, K. S. Murthy and R. U. Nesbitt, *Pharm. Tech.*, **8**, 64 (1984).

[10] T. Lindholm and M. Juslin, *Pharm. Ind.*, **44**, 937 (1982).

[11] M. Donbrow and S. Benita, *J. Pharm. Pharmacol.*, 547 (1982).

[12] J.-L. Salmon and E. Doelker, *Pharm. Acta Helv.*, **55**, 174 (1980).

[13] A. Peña Romero, M. Poncet, J. C. Jinot and D. Chulia, *Pharm. Acta Helv.*, **63**, 333 (1988)

[14] J. C. Jinot, F. Nevoux, A. Peña Romero and M. Poncet, *STP Pharma*, **5**, 12 (1989).

[15] C. Cohard, D. Chulia, Y. Gonthier and A. Verain, *Int. J. Pharm. Tech. Prod. Manuf.*, **6**, 10 (1985).

[16] A. Delacourte-Thibaut, J. C. Guyot and M. Traisnel, *Sci. Tech. Pharm.*, **11**, 131 (1982).

[17] J. C. Guyot, *Proc. 4th Int. Conf. on Pharmaceutical Technology, APGI, Paris*, Vol. 4, 1986, p. 32.

[18] P. Ozil and M. H. Rochat, *Int. J. Pharm.*, **42**, 11 (1988).

[19] O. L. Davies, *Design and Analysis of Industrial Experiments*, Oliver and Boyd, London, 1967.

[20] J. Cobby, M. Mayersohn and G. C. Walker, *J. Pharm. Sci.*, **63**, 725 (1974).

[21] F. Langenbucher, *Pharm. Ind.*, **38**, 472 (1976).

5

Analysis of different parameters of an optimized prolonged release formulation obtained by five processes

A. Peña Romero and **A. Vérain**
Université Scientifique et Médicale de Grenoble, UFR de Pharmacie–Pharmacie Galénique, Avenue de Verdun, 38243 Meylan, France
J. B. Costa
INRS, France
D. Chulia
Université de Limoges, UFR de Pharmacie–Pharmacie Galénique, 2 rue Docteur Marcland, 87025 Limoges, France
A. T. Luong
Searle de France, 52 rue Marcel Dasault, 92514 Boulogne Billancourt, France

INTRODUCTION

In previous work, a prolonged release formulation was obtained by five different processes, and it was optimized by applying a statistical strategy [1–5]:

direct compression: factorial and centred composite designs
double compression: Hadamard matrix and factorial design
compaction of the mixture of five raw materials: fractional 2^{3-1} factorial design
separate compaction of the drug and PVC: fractional 2^{5-2} factorial design
wet granulation: 3^2 design and stepwise regression

A mathematical model was found for each studied response. From the models, the contoured curves and the response surfaces were plotted, and the optimal points were sought and confirmed.

The aim of this study is to analyse and choose the best process for a formula which contains an anti-inflammatory agent (diclofenac sodium), two inert polymer matrices (PVC, ethylcellulose) and two lubricants (magnesium stearate, talc).

MATERIALS

The formula contained the following raw materials:

Diclofenac sodium	(Secifarma)	25.0%
Ethylcellulose N-7	(Hercules)	26.1%
Pevikon PE 737 P (PVC)	(SEPPIC)	45.9%
Magnesium stearate	(Prophac)	1.0%
Talc USP	(Prophac)	2.0%

For the wet granulation formulation, 2.12% Glucidex 2B (Roquette) was added as binder.

METHODS AND TESTS PERFORMED

The following responses (Y_i) and properties were studied:

(1) the powder flow rate (Y_1), the cohesion index PS/TS (Y_2), the tablet weight variation (Y_3), the friability (Y_4), the amount of drug dissolved at 8 h (Y^5) and its coefficient of variation (Y_7), the area under the dissolution curve AUC (Y^6) and its coefficient of variation (Y_8);
(2) the volume before and after tapping ($V_{10}-V_{500}$), the lubrication index (R), the ejection force (F_e), the residual force (F_r), the total energy (E_t) and the coefficient of variation of the applied upper punch force (CV UPF);
(3) the compressibility factor (f), the plasticity index (PI) and the compressibility index (Comp);
(4) the porosity factor (f_{por}) and the flowability index (ic).

Optimization will concern the following aspects:

(a) the parameters of the mathematical models,
(b) the optimized responses and evaluated properties,
(c) analysis of the data and the statistical strategies,
(d) the dissolution profiles and the fitted physical models,
(e) the processes.

The parameters of the mathematical models

The applied upper punch force (UPF) exhibited a poor influence on several optimized responses. Nevertheless, it is possible to observe that the increment of this parameter is related to adequate values of the responses. In fact, the increase of UPF value (Table 1)

Table 1 — Effect of the UPF increase on the optimized responses

Process	Y_2	Y_3	Y_4	Y_5	Y_6	Y_7	Y_8
Direct compression Frogerais	↓	↓	↓	↓	↓	↓	↓
Double compression	↓	↑	↓	↓	↓	↑ ∴	↑
Compaction of the mixture	↓	—	—	↓	↓	—	—
Separate compaction	↑	—	—	—	—	—	—
Wet granulation	↓	—	↓	↓	↓	↓	↓

(1) enhances, in general, the compression behaviour (Y_2) and the friability (Y_4),
(2) prolongs the liberation of the drug (because of the diminution of Y_5 and Y_6),
(3) diminishes the dissolution variability (Y_7 and Y_8).

The particle size range, when indicated in the model, demonstrated the most important effect on the liberation of diclofenac sodium. In the case of the separate compaction process, as the particle size range of the drug increased and the particle size range of PVC decreased, a prolonged release effect was observed [4].

The optimized responses and evaluated properties

The area under the dissolution curve (AUC=Y_6), was chosen as the major response to be optimized. Nevertheless, the results showed that it is necessary to study several properties to define the best formulation: adequate powder flow, compression behaviour and particularly, a minimal variability of the dissolution parameters [3]. It was noted that good powder flow rate is not always related to an adequate compression behaviour [4].

The coefficient of correlation values (R^2) were quite low for the estimated friability mathematical models. It seems that this response was independent of the studied parameters and their levels and, in our case, friability was not an important response to be optimized. This response could only be an evaluated property. Lindberg and Holmsquist [6] had also obtained low R^2 values for this response (R^2=0.57 and 0.68).

The analysis of the data and the statistical strategies

Our research [5,7] showed the value of the so-called '*indirect optimization designs*' [8]. The exploration of the response surfaces and the contoured curves enabled us to observe the significant number of combinations giving an optimal point. From the mathematical models, the precise experimental conditions of an optimal point could be estimated and confirmed for the major response (AUC).

A good optimization with a minimum number of experiments may be quickly reached by

(1) carrying out some preliminary trials to diminish the number of parameters,
(2) selecting the key responses by applying one of the multivariate analyses, for example principal component analysis (PCA) [9–11].
(3) defining the parameters showing a significant influence on the selected responses (ANOVA, *F* test, etc.),
(4) performing the regression on each replicate (in our case on each tablet) and not on the mean value, in order to avoid an overestimated R^2 value [3], and
(5) evaluating the R^2 value, the residual error and the lack of fit to choose the best mathematical model.

The dissolution profiles and the fitted physical models

In all the formulations, the Higuchi model parameters estimated by a non-linear regression gave the largest dispersion values (in terms of variance). This model supposes a negligible change of the tablet surface during the dissolution test [12]. In fact, the evaluated tablets exhibited, in general, a partial or total disintegration after 14 h, which explains the worst fit.

With the exception of the formulation obtained by direct compression in a rotary machine, the dissolution profiles were well fitted by the Weibull function. A high density in the centre of the tablets may explain the sigmoid dissolution profiles. A percentage of the drug remains imprisoned in the matrix after the dissolution test. It is possible to suppose that, in the densified central zone of the tablet, the diameters of the pores are smaller than the diameters of the drug particles covered by the inert polymers.

The processes

Table 2 contains the pertinent information about the evaluated responses and properties previously described. The optimal values are given to compare the processes.

When compared with direct compression results, the dry granulation processes enhance the flow of the powder and decrease the variability of the AUC, the major response. Nevertheless, this variability and the variability of the drug dissolved at 8 h (Y_7) are greater than the fixed optimal values, particularly for the compaction processes. From the results it is seen that the wet granulation process gave a powder presenting an adequate or better result than the other processes:

powder flow rate (Y_1)>10 g^{-1}/s;
cohesion index (Y_2<100;
variability values of the tablet weight (Y_3), of the dissolution parameters (Y_7, Y_8) and of the UPF lower than the fixed limits; moreover, only the wet granulation process results in a dissolution variability <5%;
adequate values for the lubrication index (R), F_c and F_r;
small E_t value and applied UPF (7 kN);
good compressibility;
optimal plasticity index.

Table 2 — Optimized process results

Response	Direct compression Betapress	Double compression	Compaction of the mixture	Separate compaction	Wet granulation	Optimal value
Y_1 (g^{-1}/s)	0	11.11	16.7	13.0	13.2	>10
Y_2	71	92	112	165	73	>100
Y_3 (CV, %)	1.8	0.58	0.33	0.68	0.41	<1
Y_4 (%)	0.09	0.51	0.40	0.62	1.02	<1
Y_5 (%)	56.5	69.9	73	66.0	75.9	near 60
Y_6 (% h)	667	701	736	722	717	near 713
Y_7 (CV, %)	12.4	8.3	16.5	15.9	4.3	<5
Y_8 (CV, %)	9.0	4.9	5.6	8.7	3.0	<5
Y_{10}-V_{500} (mL)	52	10	27	15	24	<20
R	0.82	0.89	0.88	0.96	0.92	near 1.0
F_c (kN)	0.21	0.18	0.13	0.14	0.17	minimal
F_r (kN)	0.17	0.09	0.19	0.04	0.07	minimal
E_t (N m)	33.5	27.54	66.3	38.2	24	minimal
CV UPF (%)	4.0	3.83	2.6	3.6	1.05	<2
f (%)	28.3	5.6	10.0	12.6	10.7	5–8
PI (%)	93.0	91.5	78.3	83.3	94.1	100
C_{omp} (%)	49.8	16.3	5.0	7.2	25.4	near 100
f_{por} (%)	28.8	23.7	16.6	21.8	32.8	<50
ic	4.5	6.7	5.4	5.4	3.5	>10

EXPERIMENTAL TESTS ON THE OPTIMIZED FORMULATIONS: SEEKING THE BEST PROCESS

At this stage, we wanted to answer the following questions.

(1) Is the flowability test sensitive to the technological change of the same optimized formula?
(2) Is porosity associated with the dissolution profile, and with one of the studied parameters?
(3) As the AUC value is almost the same, may the β parameter of the Weibull function be used for evaluating the variability between tablets and between processes?

The flowability test

The flowability test was carried out in a Jenike cell [3,13].

The flow function illustrated in Fig. 1 reveals a singular behaviour of the powders which may be associated with the process or with the high percentage of PVC. In fact, even if the curves were obtained by linear regression, a marked dispersion may be

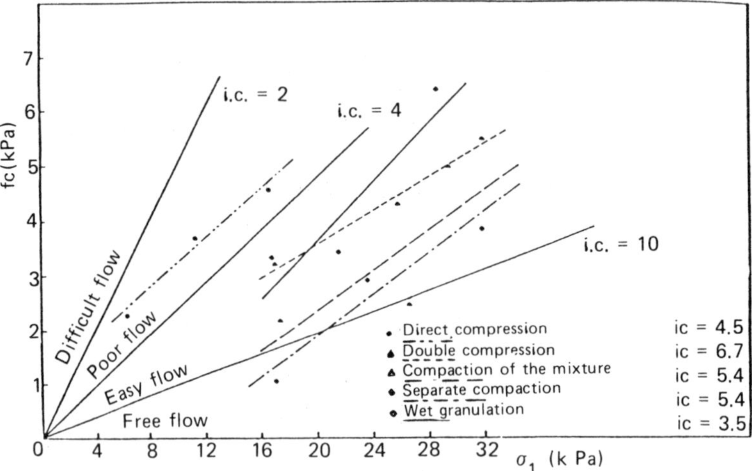

Fig. 1 — Flow function and flowability (ic) of the optimized formulations.

seen, particularly for the compaction of the mixture and, curiously, for the wet granulation powder.

Regarding the flow function values, powders may be classed in two groups:

(1) the direct compression powder, representing poor flow;
(2) the granulated powders, giving easy flow.

Because of this singular behaviour of the powders, it was supposed that the powder blends were not homogeneous even though the variability of the tablet weight was at a minimum. This means that the test is very sensitive to the technological modifications of the same formula.

The porosimetry measurements

In order to characterize the microstructure of the matrices, the total porosimetry factor, the pore volume, the pore surface and the mean pore diameter were measured using a mercury porosimeter (Micrometrics) [3]. The mean of three replicates and their coefficient of variation are indicated in Table 3.

From the results, it is possible to draw the following conclusions.

(1) In accordance with the Dubinin classification [14], all the matrix tablets exhibited macropores (mean pore diameter >200Å).
(2) The tablets obtained by direct compression in a single punch machine (Frogerais) and those obtained by wet granulation had very similar values; only the coefficient of variation differentiate these two processes.
(3) As expected, as the applied UPF increased, the porosimetry parameters decreased (UPF values: direct compression and wet granulation, 7 kN; double

Table 3 — Porosimetry measurements

Process	Parameter	Porosity factor (%)	Pore volume ($cm^3 g^{-1}$)	Pore surface $m^2 g^{-1}$)	Mean pore diameter[a] (μm)
Direct compression in Betapress	Mean	28.8	0.269	33.00	0.152
	CV	6.1	9.3	16.2	26.85
Direct compression in Frogerais	Mean	33.8	0.336	34.40	0.23
	CV	2.1	3.3	6.5	11.5
Double compression	Mean	23.7	0.207	34.14	0.068
	CV	2.8	2.8	4.0	4.2
Compaction of the mixture	Mean	16.6	0.132	31.21	0 .022
	CV	3.9	3.7	4.6	4.5
Separate compaction	Mean	21.8	0.184	32.09	0.057
	CV	6.0	7.1	3.8	17.4
Wet granulation	Mean	32.8	0.311	33.82	0.252
	CV	1.9	2.6	1.6	6.4

[a]Pore diameter when cumulative volume is 50%.

compression, 12 kN; separate compaction, 19 kN; compaction of the mixture, 31 kN).

(4) The variability of the porosity parameters may be used to differentiate the processes. It also explains the variability of the dissolution parameters because of the same order of variation (CV):

wet granulation (3.0)<double compression (4.9)<compaction of the mixture (5.6)<separate compaction (8.7)<direct compression (9.0)

Three important aspects may be cited when interpreting the pore size distributions (Fig. 2).

(1) For an applied mercury pressure of 0–30 000 lbf in^{-2} (absolute), the mean pore diameter varies from 391 to 0.006 μm.
(2) It is easy to observe the important effect of UPF: the pore size distributions tend to go to the right as UPF increases; this means that, for the same accumulated intrusion volume, the mean pore diameter is smaller as UPF increases.

In accordance with the growing UPF values, the pore size distributions are more to the right in the following order:

Process	*UPF* (kN)
Wet granulation	7
Direct compression in Frogerais	7

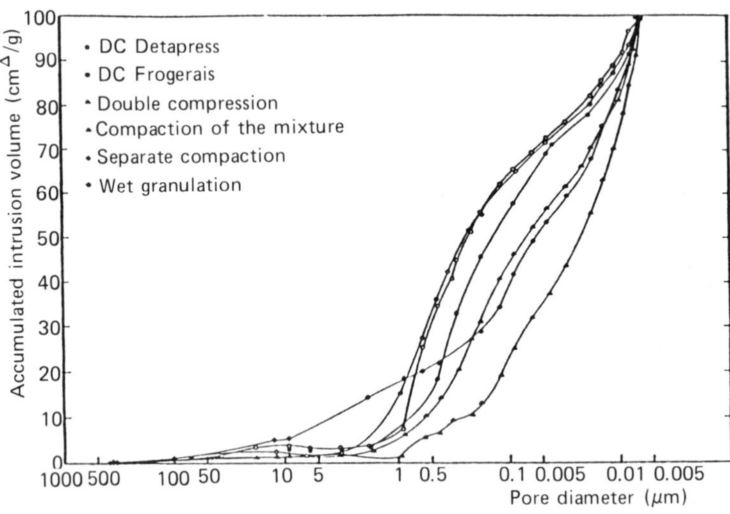

Fig. 2 — The pore size distributions of the optimized tablets.

Direct compression on Betapress	7
Double compression	12
Separate compaction	19
Compaction of the mixture	31

From the analysis, it is possible to suppose that the UPF applied on the Betapress rotary machine must be found between 7 and 12 kN.

(3) The effect of UPF is verified by observing the similar pore size distributions of the wet granulation and the direct compression tablets in Frogerais, after 25% of the cumulative volume.

Therefore the pore size distribution seems to be dependent on the applied compression force rather than the process, when the formula and the area under the dissolution curve were kept constant.

Comparison fo the dissolution profiles

Estimated F_∞ and β parameters from the Weibull Function

The estimated F_∞ and β parameters are given in Table 4.

The double compression process results in significant retention of the drug in the inert matrix 14 h after the dissolution test (F_∞=0.87).

Fig. 3 illustrates the effect of the process on the same formula and for near AUC values. The wet granulation release profile exhibits a marked sigmoid aspect owing to the high β value.

Table 4 — Estimates F_∞ and β parameters

Process	F_∞	β
Direct compression on Betapress	1.0	1.51
Direct compression on Frogerais	0.96	1.65
Double compression	0.87	2.46
Compaction of the mixture	0.94	2.68
Separate compaction	0.95	2.03
Wet granulation	0.92	3.38

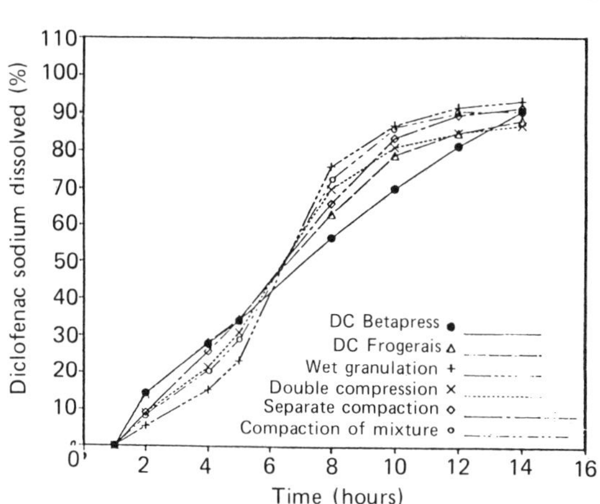

Fig. 3 — Effect of the process on the release profiles.

Analysis of covariance

The analysis of covariance between a continuous variable (β is the curve shape parameter from the Weibull function) and a discrete variable (process) was determined using the general linear model (GLM) procedure from the Statistical Analysis System (SAS). The technique of the heterogeneity of slopes showed that there was no significant difference (Tables 5 and 6).

Table 5 — R^2 and β values

	Direct compression on Betapress	Direct compression on Frogerais	Double compression	Compaction of the mixture	Separate compaction	Wet granulation
R^2	0.97	0.98	0.97	0.95	0.98	0.96
β	1.51	1.65	2.46	2.68	2.03	3.38

Table 6 — Slope comparisons between processes (p values)

Direct compression on Betapress vs. direct compression on Frogerais	0.148	NS
Direct compression on Betapress vs. double compression	<0.001	***
Direct compression on Betapress vs. compaction of the mixture	<0.001	***
Direct compression on Betapress vs. separate compaction	<0.001	***
Direct compression on Betapress vs.wet granulation	<0.001	***
Direct compression on Frogerais vs. double compression	<0.001	***
Direct compression on Frogerais vs. compaction of the mixture	0.001	**
Direct compression on Frogerais vs. separate compaction	0.010	*
Direct compression on Frogerais vs. wet granulation	<0.001	***
Double compression vs. compaction of the mixture	<0.294	NS
Double compression vs. separater compaction	0.021	*
Double compression vs. wet granulation	<0.001	***
Compaction of the mixture vs. separate compaction	0.019	*
Compaction of the mixture vs. wet granulation	0.029	*
Separate compaction vs. wet granulation	0.001	***

Significance: NS, none; ***, high; **, regular; *, poor.

(1) between the two direct compression processes performed in a single-punch machine (β=1.51) and in rotary machine (β=1.65), or
(2) between the formula obtained by compaction by the five raw materials (β=2.68) and the formula obtained by double compression (β=2.46).

As the other comparisons between slopes are significant (p<0.05), the β parameter may help to differentiate one process from another if the optimization experimental conditions are kept constant. There was no significant difference between trials in all the processes, indicating that dissolution values (in terms of β) can be reproduced (Table 7).

Table 7 — Variability between trials and between tablets (p values)

	Direct compression on Betapress	Direct compression on Frogerais	Double compression	Compaction of the mixture	Separate compaction	Wet granulation
Between trials	0.08	−0.954	−0.576	0.16		
Between tablets	<0.001***	0.118	0.959	0.374	0.008**	0.99

Significance: **, regular; ***, high.

A significant difference was found between tablets for the formulations obtained by direct compression in a rotary machine and by separate compaction.

Principal Component Analysis (PCA)

The objective of PCA is to obtain a small number of linear combinations (the principal components) representative of the entire system [3,9–11]. The summarized information is evaluated by the percentage of the total variance justified by the component.

In our study, we only retained two components, obtained by the analysis on each tablet of the optimized formulations:

Principal component	*Proportion of variance (%)*	*Cumulative proportion (%)*
1	53.9	53.9
2	32.2	86.1

The plot of the two components (Fig. 4) reveals the following points.

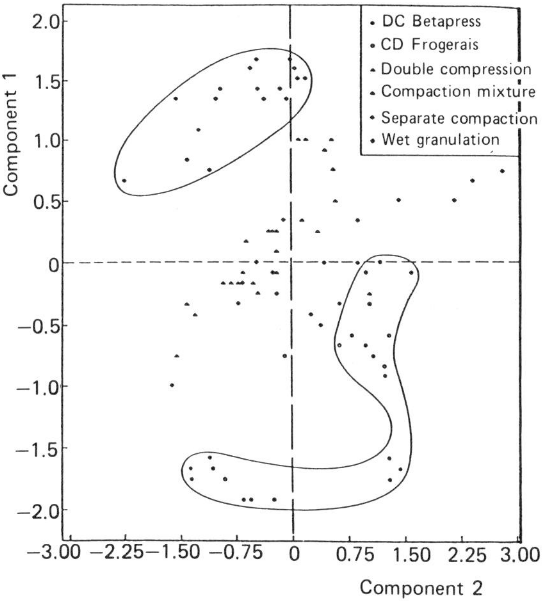

Fig. 4 — The principal component analysis.

(1) The first component, which expresses the curve shape, exhibits an 'opposition' of the release profiles obtained by wet granulation and by direct compression. The wet granulation profile has a sigmoid aspect while the direct compression profiles, particularly those for the tablets obtained in rotary machine, are nearly linear.

(2) The second component, which expresses the mean level of dissolution, cannot discriminate between the release profiles. This is explained by the similar AUC

values of the formulations. In addition, we noted that AUC is a linear combination of the time (T_i) as the second component.

(3) A high variability between tablets is observed for the direct compression and for the separate compaction, owing to the largest dispersion of the corresponding points.

Discriminant analysis

A discriminant analysis was also applied with the aim of obtaining the linear combinations of T_i (time) discriminating the processes.

While PCA searches for the linear combinations containing the total variation, discriminant analysis searches for the linear combinations containing or 'explaining' the variation between processes.

In the plot of the first components (Fig. 5), the difference between the wet granulation and the direct compression profiles is confirmed. The first component discriminates between the shape profiles. The second component discriminates between the initial slopes of the release profiles. Then, it is possible to differentiate between the separate compaction and the other processes, because it has the highest initial slope. This is also observed in Fig. 3.

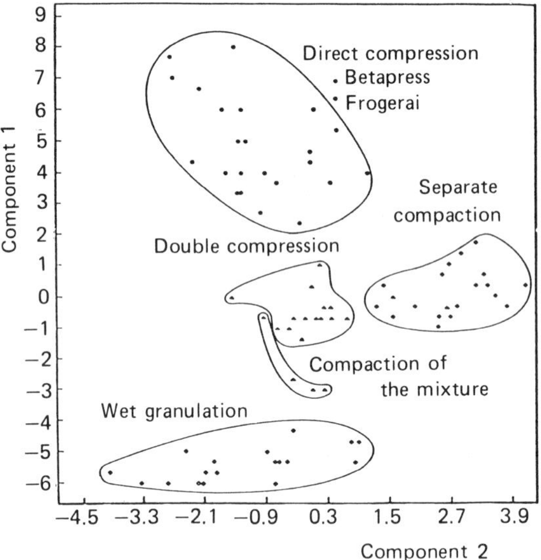

Fig. 5 — Discriminant analysis.

CONCLUSION

The work previously performed [5,7] shows the importance of experimental design for reaching an optimized formulation with a minimum number of experiments.

From experimental testing of this work we could arrive at the following conclusions.

(1) The flowability test in a Jenike cell was very sensitive to the technological modifications of the same optimized formulation; therefore, it can be used for quality control during the development, scale-up or production of medicaments.
(2) The variability of the porosity parameters may be used to differentiate between the processes and to explain the variability of the dissolution parameters.
(3) There was no significant difference between trials in all the processes, indicating that dissolution values can be reproducible; the β parameter may help to differentiate one process from another and to evaluate the variability between trials and between tablets.

The plots of two components obtained from PCA and from discriminant analysis, revealed an 'opposition' between tablets obtained by wet granulation and by direct compression. In fact, the principal component represents the curve shape of the dissolution profiles (β), which, in these two processes, were quite different.

The Higuchi model gave the worst fit for the data because of the change of the tablet surface during the dissolution test. With the exception of the formulation obtained by direct compression in a rotary machine, the dissolution profiles were well fitted by the Weibull function. A high density in the centre of the tablets may explain the sigmoid aspect of the dissolution profiles.

In terms of the flow properties, the physics of compression, the variability of the dissolution and porosimetry parameters and the variability between trials, the wet granulated formula showed best results in almost all cases. This process is then proposed for the study of prolonged release formulations.

ACKNOWLEDGEMENTS

The authors would like to thank CONACYT, Mexico, FESC–UNAM, Mexico, CEFI, Paris and Searle, France, for their support of this study.

REFERENCES

[1] A. Peña Romero, M. Poncet, J. C. Jinot and D. Chulia, *Pharm. Acta Helv.*, **63**, 333 (1988).
[2] A. Peña Romero, J. B. Costa, I. Castel-Maroteaux and D. Chulia, *Proc. 8th Pharmaceutical Technology Conf. Monte Carlo,* Vol. 2, 1989, p. 64.
[3] A. Peña Romero, *Ph.D. Thesis*, University of Grenoble I, France, 1989.
[4] A. Peña Romero, J. B. Costa, D. Chulia and A. T. Luong, *Proc. 5th Int. Conf. on Pharmaceutical Technology, APGI, Paris*, Vol. 4, 1989, p. 174.
[5] A. Piña Romero, J. B. Costa, J. C. Jinot and D. Chulia, *Proc. 5th Int. Conf. on Pharmnaceutical Technology, APGI, Paris*, Vol. 5, 1989, p. 380.
[6] N-O. Lindberg and B. Holmsquist, *Drug Dev. Ind. Pharm.*, **13**, 1063 (1987).

[7] J. C. Jinot, F. Nevoux, A. Peña Romero and M. Poncet, *STP Pharma,* **5** 12 (1989).
[8] R. Roufffiac, M., Magbi, F. Rodríguez, N. Benkaddour and L. Bonnet, *J. Pharm. Belg.,* **42**, 5 (1987).
[9] N. R. Bohidat, F. A. Restaino and J. B. Schwartz, *J. Pharm. Sci.,* **64**, 966 (1975).
[10] P. Wehrle, P. Nobelis, S. I. Saleh and A. Stamm, *Proc. 8th Pharmaceutical Technology Conf., Monte Carlo*, Vol. 1, 1989, p. 164.
[11] P. Wehrle, P. Nobelis and A. Stamm, *STP Pharma,* **4**, 275 (1988).
[12] T. Higuchi, *J. Pharm. Sci.,* **52**, 1145 (1963).
[13] Y. Gonthier and D. Chulia-Clement, *Proc. 3rd Int. Conf. on Pharmaceutical Technology, APGI, Paris,* Vol. 1, 1983, p. 37.
[14] M. M. Dubinin, *Pure Appl. Chem.,* **10**, 309 (1965).

6

Controlled release matrix tablets of ketoprofen

Paola Mura and **Giampiero Bramanti**
Department of Pharmaceutical Sciences, Via G. Capponi 9, Firenze, Italy
Luca Fabbri
Pharmaceutical Technology Laboratory, Menarini SaS, Via Sette Santi 3, Firenze, Italy
Maurizio Valleri
Pharmaceutical Technology Laboratory, Malesci SpA, Via Paisiello 8, Firenze, Italy

SUMMARY

To obtain a prolonged action dosage form of ketoprofen, three different techniques for delaying drug release from hydrophilic matrices of hydroxypropylmethylcellulose were evaluated. They were incorporation of glyceryl monostearate, as a release controller, partial coating with an impermeable covering of cellulose acetate phthalate, and pan-spray coating with a mixture of insoluble (Eudragit) and soluble (PEG 400) polymers. The *in vitro* release profiles of each formulation were studies using the USP basket method. Pan-spray coating with the Eudragit–PEG mixture was found to be the best technique, enabling the desired release profile to be obtained through variation of the coating thickness.

INTRODUCTION

Ketoprofen (2-(3-benzoylphenyl)propionic acid), one of the most active non-steroidal anti-inflammatory drugs, is employed in the long-term treatment of rheumatoid arthritis and also as an analgesic in the treatment of pain of varying origins [1]. Clinical use, however, requires a dose schedule of 100–200 mg 3–4 times a day, the duration of action of a single oral dose being only 6–8 h [2].

Development of a prolonged action dosage form of ketoprofen will bring about several desirable therapeutic advantages: improvement of patient compliance;

minimization of blood level fluctuations; reduction of the total amount of drug administered; reduction of incidence of both local and systemic adverse side effects [3].

The aim of this investigation was to create a sustained release dosage form to provide a constant blood level pattern for up to 12h after oral administration of ketoprofen. Three different techniques for delaying drug release from hydrophilic matrices of hydroxyproplmethylcellulose were evaluated.

EXPERIMENTAL

Materials

Ketoprofen (SIMS), hydroxypropylmethylcellulose E5 (HPMC, η=2%, 5mPa s, Dow Chemical), glyceryl monostearate (Precirol, Gattefossè), Eudragit E 30 D (Rhom Pharma), Polyethylene glycol 400 (PEG 400, Merck) and cellulose acetate phthalate (CAP, Ambrochim) were used directly without any prior purification.

Systems preparation

Hydrophilic matrices

These were prepared with HPMC as a matrix agent and magnesium stearate as a lubricant, according to the following formula: ketoprofen, 110mg; HPMC, 488mg; Mg stearate, 2mg. The powders were mixed after sieving (300 μm) the single components, and the flow properties of the mixture were controlled. The tablets (KET-R) were manufactured on a Korsch rotary tableting machine. The hardness of the tablets was measured on a Schleuniger model 2E hardness tester.

Hydrophilic matrices containing Precirol

Varying amounts of Precirol in Precirol: drug ratios of 1:3 (KET-R A), 1:2 (KET-R B) and 1:1 (KET-R C) were added to the above formulation for hydrophilic matrices. The properties of these tablets are shown in Table 1 (average of 20 measurements).

Table 1 — Properties of the tablets

Tablet	Mass (mg±SD)	Drug content (mg±SD)	Hardness (kPa)	Thickness (mm±SD)
KET-R	603±3.8	112±1.5	12	6.6±0.08
KET-R A	614±5.7	109±1.6	6	6.5±0.10
KET-R B	649±6.8	111±1.8	9	7.1±0.05
KET-R C	702±7.0	109±2.4	9	7.5±0.02

Partially coated tablets

The surface of KET-R cores was 2/3 coated by careful immersion in CAP acetone-saturated solution (KET-R CAP tablets).

Coated tablets

The surface of KET-R cores was pan coated with a mixture having the following composition: Eudragit 'E30 D', 50%; PEG 400, 2%; talc, 2%; deionized water, 46%. Talc was included as an antiagglomerating agent in order to prevent stickiness during the coating process [4]. Tablets with three different polymer film thicknesses (6, 10 and 15 mg) were prepared (KET-R, 10 and 15). The hardness of all coated tablets was greater than 25 kp.

The finished tablets prepared were stored for 24 h at 20°C before the release tests.

Release experiments

The release tests were performed using the USP dissolution method (apparatus I) and utilized 1000 ml of pH 1.2 simulated gastric fluid (USP XXI) or pH 6.8 simulated intestinal fluid (USP XXI) without enzymes, equilibrated to 37°C and stirred with the basket rotating at 50 or 150 rev/min. Drug concentrations were assayed by UV spectrophotometry at 255 nm. The experiments were continued until 100% dissolution was achieved. The release data were analysed to zero order, calculating the slope and intercept of the line. Each data point is the average of six individual determinations. In all cases the standard deviation was less than 9%.

Core volume measurements (hydration and erosion)

The diminution in volume of glassy core was measured with a penetrometer [5] calibrated at 0.01 mm with a 0.5 mm diameter pin, determining the position of the glassy–rubbery interface (swelling front) relative to the initial height and diameter of the glassy core. At fixed intervals during the dissolution test the system was withdrawn from the basket and placed under the penetrometer pin in a horizonal or vertical position; then the pin was dipped into the swollen layer until the glassy core was reached (swelling front). The reductions in height and diameter were measured; then the volume change of the glassy core was calculated, plotted vs. time and fitted using a straight-line equation.

RESULTS AND DISCUSSION

The proper dose of ketoprofen for an optimized zero-order model to obtain the desired drug level pattern to remain in the therapeutic range for 12 h (twice-a-day formulation) was estimated from drug pharmacokinetic parameters [6] by conventional equations [3] on the basis of a one-compartment open model and was found to be 110 mg.

The use of cellulose ethers in producing matrix-type sustained release tablets is well documented [7]. Hydrophilic matrices of ketoprofen with hydroxypropylmethylcellulose (KET-R) were manufactured by direct compression. This allowed reproducibility of the core substrate avoiding granulation and its related variables (constant characteristics of granulated, residual moisture, etc.).

The release curve of ketoprofen obtained from the KET-R tablet at pH 1.2 and 50 rev/min is shown in Fig. 1. The release profile was zero order up to 90% drug content. The equation obtained by plotting the percentage released vs. time was $y=0.187x-1.997$, $r=0.99$. No burst effect was present.

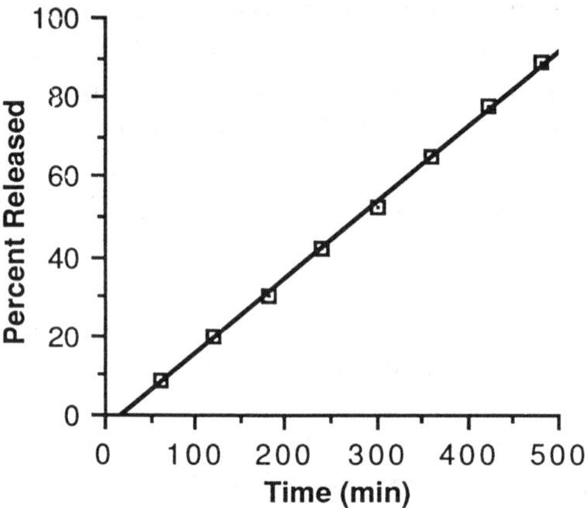

Fig. 1 — Release profile of ketoprofen from tablet KET-R; basket 50 rev/min; pH 1.2.

The effect of basket rotation rate and pH on the release profile of ketoprofen from the KET-R tablet is presented in Fig. 2. The release rate of ketoprofen from the

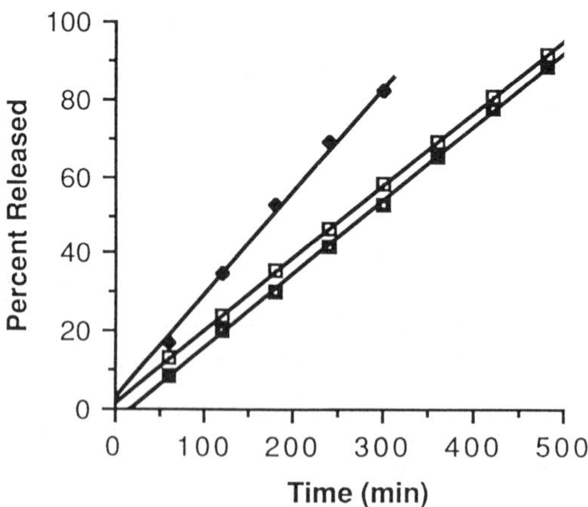

Fig. 2 — Effect of basket rotation rate and of pH on the release profile of ketoprofen from tablets KET-R: ■, 50 rev/min, pH 1.2; □, 50 rev/min, pH 6.8; ◆, 150 rev/min, pH 1.2.

system increased with increasing basket rotation rate and changed from 11%/h at 50 rev/min to 16%/h at 150 rev/min, but the profile remained linear up to 80% drug content. Moreover, the drug release profile at pH 6.8 (y=0.189x−1.091, r=0.99) was very similar to that at pH 1.2 and thus the ketoprofen released from such a matrix tablet was practically independent of pH. The glassy core volume decrease was linear, as Fig. 3 shows, and the decrease rate was greater at pH 1.2 (20.363 mm^3/min) than at pH 6.8 (12.985 mm^3/min), even though it does not influence the drug release rate. Therefore this drug delviery system can be considered to follow a constant drug

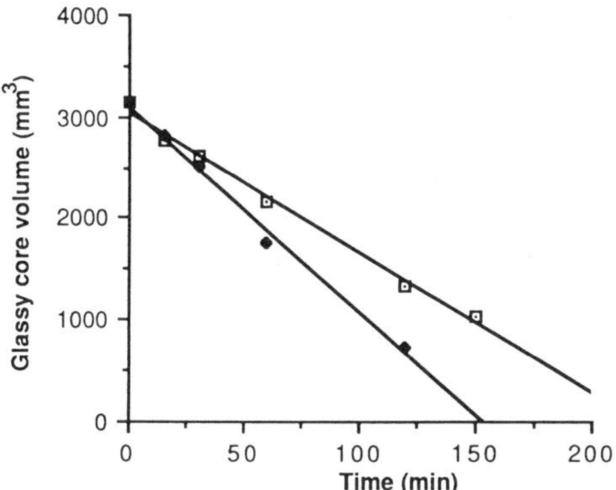

Fig. 3 — Glassy core volume decrease of tablets KET-R vs. time: ◆, pH 1.2; ⊡, pH 6.8.

release. However, in spite of these positive characteristics, the drug release rate from KET-R tablets was to high for the desired twice-daily formulation to be obtained. Three different techniques for delaying drug release from these cores were then evaluated:

(a) incorporation of a release retardant such as Precirol;
(b) coating of 2/3 core surface with an impermeable covering by careful immersion in CAP;
(c) a new approach based on pan-spray coating with a mixture of insoluble (Eudragit E 30D) and soluble (PEG 400) polymers.

Precirol was successfully used as a retardant in matrix tablet formulations [8]. The effect of Precirol incorporation into the hydroxypropylmethylcellulose matrix tablets was therefore investigated. Precirol: drug ratios of 1:3, 1:2 and 1:1 were used (tablets KET-R A, B, and C). No significant differences in the volume decrease profiles of glassy cores and in ketoprofen release profiles (Fig. 4) in comparison with original core were obtained, even with increased Precirol.

In order to reduce further the ketoprofen release rate from matrix tablets, the partial coating of the cores with CAP was assayed. This technique was successfully applied to obtain a progammable zero-order drug delivery system [5].

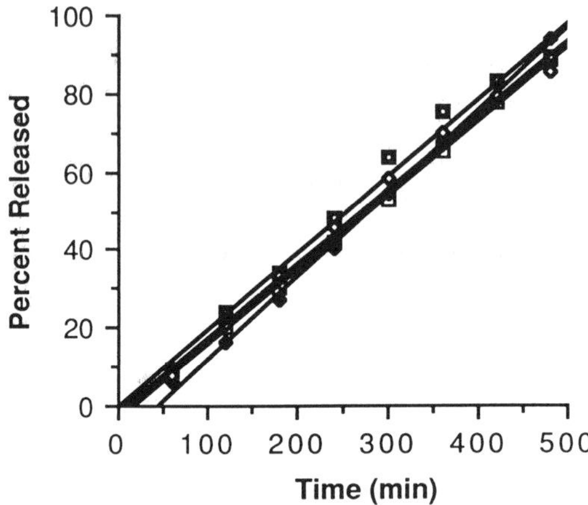

Fig. 4 — Release profile of ketoprofen from tablets containing Precirol (50 rev/min; pH 1.2): ⊡, tablet KET-R; ◆, tablet KET-R A; ■, tablet KET-R B; ◆, tablet KET-R C.

The release profile of ketoprofen from the 2/3 CAP coated core (KET-R CAP tablet) was of zero order (y=0.037x−1.263, r=0.99) and the drug release rate was clearly lower than the original core, as is shown in Fig. 5. However, the technique of preparation of KET-R CAP tablets was somewhat complex, requiring considerable accuracy in the partial coating phase, and not easily applicable on an industrial scale.

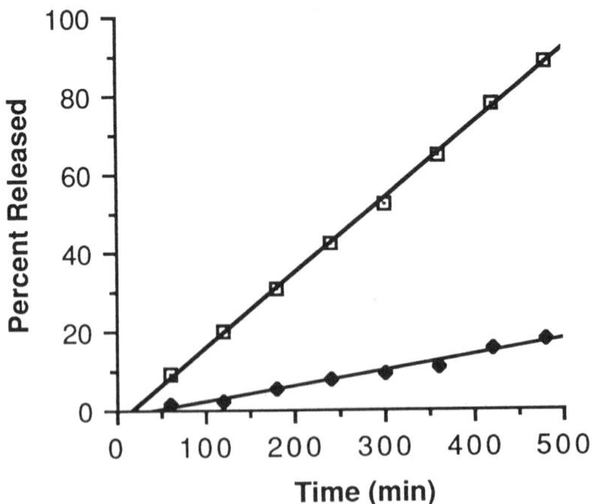

Fig. 5 — Release profile of ketoprofen from tablet 2/3 CAP coated (50 rev/min; pH 1.2): ◆, tablet KET-R; ⊡, tablet KET-R CAP.

In view of the above results a new approach based on core panspray coating was experimented with a mixture of Eudragit E 30D and PEG 400 was chosen as a coating: Eudragit, completely insoluble in water, was the retardant, while PEG 400 was added in order to form ionophorous pores, thus allowing the drug release rate to be controlled.

Tablets coated with the Eudragit–PEG 400 mixture were made with three different polymer film thicknesses: 6, 10 and 15 mg (KET-R, 10 and 15 tablets). For these tablets it was not possible to obtain swelling measurements because this was prevented by the lake coating.

The ketoprofen release profiles from these tablets are shown in Fig. 6. The

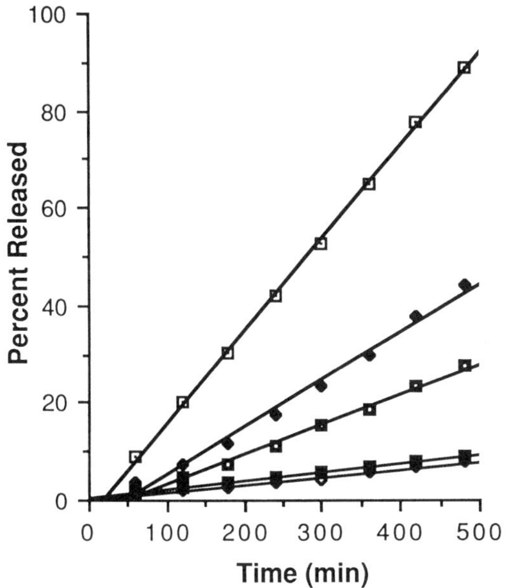

Fig. 6 — Release profile of ketoprofen from Eudragit-PEG 400 coated tablets (50 rev/min; pH 1.2): ⊡, tablet KET-R 6; ■, tablet KET-R 10; ◇, tablet KET-R 15; ■, Orudis retard.

release curves were linear (r=0.99) and the release rate appeared to decrease with increasing coating amounts. On the basis of the linear inverse relation found between the drug release rate and the coat (Fig. 7), the release rate can be varied with predictable effects by varying the coating amount. In particular the KET-R 15 tablet showed a lower rate of drug release than the 2/3 CAP coated tablet (0.96%/h instead of 2.2%/h) and its release profile was similar to that of commercial sustained release capsules of ketoprofen (Orudis Retard®, 150 mg).

CONCLUSIONS

Of the techniques examined for delaying drug release from hydrophilic matrices of HPMC, only Precirol incorporation proved ineffective.

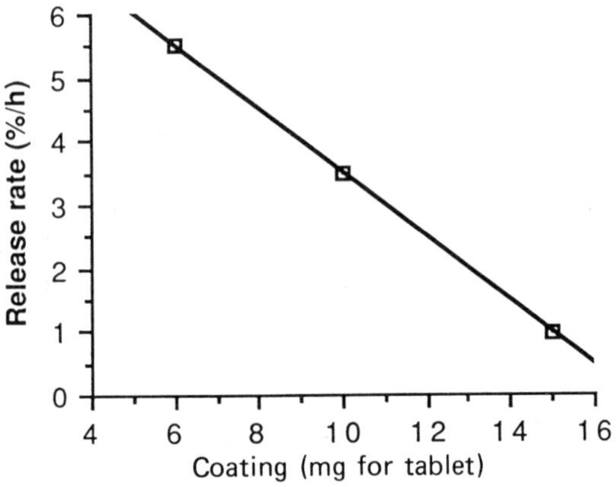

Fig. 7 — Effect of Eudragit: PEG 400 coats.

Partial coating with CAP enabled the desired decrease to be obtained, but the technique was rather complex and caused difficulties for industrial production.

Pan coating with a Eudragit–PEG 400 mixture proved to be best technique. The relative ease of manufacture and the variety of release profiles attainable make pan coating with a Eudragit E 30D–PEG 400 mixture a useful technique for obtaining sustained release tablets. Further studies will be necessary to assess the influence of Eudragit: PEG ratio on ketoprofen release characteristics.

ACKNOWLEDGEMENTS

The authors thank Mr. C. Baccani, Mr. P. Bucci and Mr. L. Ceccarelli for their technical assistance.

REFERENCES

[1] S. A. Cooper, S. Gelb, E. H. Goldman, P. Cohn and B. Cavaliere, *Clin. Pharmacol. Ther.*, **33**, 195 (1983).
[2] G. L. Craig and W. W. Buchanan, *Drugs*, **20**, 453 (1980).
[3] N. G. Lordi, in L. Lachman, H. A. Lieberman and J. L. Kanig (eds), *The Theory and Practice of Industrial Pharmacy*, Lea & Febiger, Philadelphia, PA, 6th edn, 1986, p. 430.
[4] A. M. Mehta, *Pharm. Manuf.*, **3** 27 (1986).
[5] P. Colombo, A. Gazzaniga, C. Caramella, U. Conte and A. La Manna, *Acta Pharm. Technol.*, **33**, 15 (1987).
[6] A. Goodman Gilman, L. S. Goodman, T. W. Rall and F. Murad, *The Pharmacological Basis of Therapeutics*, Macmillan, New York, 7th edn., 1985, p. 158.
[7] P. Buti, in P. Buri, F. Puisieux, E. Doelker and J. P. Benoit (eds), *Formes Pharmaceutiques Nouvelles*, Tec & Doc (Lavoisier), Paris, 1985, p. 202.
[8] S. Bolton and D. Saraiya, *Joint Japan–United States Congr. of Pharmaceutical Sciences, Honolulu, HI, 2–7 December, 1987.*

7

A new ibuprofen pulsed release oral dosage form

U. Conte
Department of Pharmaceutical Chemistry, University of Pavia, Italy
P. Columbo
Institute of Pharmaceutical Technology, University of Parma, Italy
A. La Manna
Department of Pharmaceutical Chemistry, University of Pavia, Italy
A. Gazzaniga
Institute of Pharmaceutical Chemistry, University of Milano, Italy
M. E. Sangalli and **P. Giunchedi**
Department of Pharmaceutical Chemistry, University of Pavia, Italy

SUMMARY

Constant release is not always the desired solution for controlled drug administration; some therapeutic situations require consecutive pulses. A biphasic oral delivery system able to release an immediate dose of therapeutic agent as well as a further pulse of drug after some hours would, useful. In order to obtain such a desired release performance, a new system (three-layer tablet) has been designed with the following characteristics:

(1) an energy source, able to deliver the two divided doses of drug;
(2) a control element, between the drug layers, able to delay the release of the second dose of drug, which acts as a barrier and is made with a mixture of water-swellable polymers;
(3) an outer film, which is made of water-impermeable polymer, that covers the second dose of drug and the barrier.

The new system works through subsequent interactions of aqueous fluids with the three different layers of material in the following order:

(1) rapid interaction of the uncoated part of the system, and immediate disintegration of the first dose;

(2) slow interaction of the barrier and its gelation;
(3) interaction of the second drug layer and development of a force able to break the barrier, thus promoting the release of the second dose of drug.

Preliminary *in vivo* experiments carried out on this biphasic pulsed release device containing ibuprofen as a model drug reveal two distinct peaks in plasma profiles, thus indicating that the *in vitro* results are in good agreement with the *in vivo* blood levels.

INTRODUCTION

Some new oral drug delivery systems have been prepared in previous years by our group.

(i) A 'reservoir' system consisting of a core containing the active principle and an external compressed polymeric layer [1,2].
(ii) A multiple-unit 'hybrid' reservoir system consisting of minimatrices, whose drug release is governed by the swellable properties of the polymeric core and by the thickness of the outer permeable membrane obtained by surface cross-linking or by spray coating [3–6].
(iii) An *in vitro* programmable system, a matrix with a constant releasing area, which is the main control element of the drug release. In this system the kinetics of the release is also dependent on the swelling and dissolution characteristics of the polymeric material and the influence of the solubility of the active principle is also reduced [7,8].

A further development of this system has been the preparation of drug delivery systems whereby the releasing area exposed has been reduced by an impermeable partial coating. As a result, the kinetics of release was zero order [9,10].

Frequently, the constant release of a drug from pharmaceutical dosage forms enables one to obtain a suitable pharmacological and therapeutic response. However, for therapy of certain pathologies, i.e. some heart and rheumatic diseases, or in the utilization of some drugs such as contraceptive steroids and antibiotics, it would be more useful to obtain different plasma levels of the active principle at different times related to painful symptoms or circadian rhythms, etc. In these cases the desired therapeutic results can usually be obtained with frequent administration of conventional dosage forms which lead to a prompt absorption of the active principle. This kind of drug treatment is often compromised by a lack of full compliance by the patient. Until now there have been few systems that allow the release of the active principle in successive pulses at precise and well-controlled time periods [11,12].

Taking all these considerations into account, the aim of this work was to design and prepare a new pulsed release oral drug delivery system, capable of releasing an immediate dose of drug as well as a further dose after some hours.

To obtain such a pulsed released pattern, a system based on a three-layer tablet with the following characteristics has been designed.

(1) Two layers each containing a dose of the drug.
(2) An intermediate layer acting as a control element, which separates the drug layers. This control element, made from a mixture of water-swellable

polymers, would act as a barrier in order to delay the release of the dose of the drug present in the second layer.

(3) An outer film made of an impermeable polymer (container), which coats the barrier and the second dose of the drug.

(4) An energy source, based on a fast swelling polymer, able to promote the delivery of the two doses of the drug.

Therefore, we prepared and tested compressed three-layer tablets, covered on all surfaces, except for one part of the first dose, with an impermeable coating. We employed ibuprofen as a model drug, hydroxypropylmethylcelluloses as components of the control barrier and some *superdisintegrants* as the energy source [13].

The feasibility, the *in vitro* release profiles and the *in vivo* results of some of these systems are described and discussed.

EXPERIMENTAL

Materials and methods

ibuprofen (USP XXI grade; Francis, Milano, Italy).
Corn starch (USP XXI grade; C. Erba, Milano, Italy).
Methylcellulose (500–600 cps; BDH, Poole, UK).
Ethylcellulose (22 cps; BDH, Poole, UK).
Mannitol (USP XXI grade; C. Erba, Milano, Italy).
Talc (USP XXI grade; C. Erba, Milano, Italy).
Hydroxypropylmethylcellulose (Methocel K4M and Methocel K15M; Colorcon, Orpington, UK).
Polyvinylpyrrolidone (Plasdone K 29–32, GAF Corp., New York, USA).
Magnesium stearate (USP XXI grade; C. Erba, Milano, Italy).
Sodium starch glycollate (Primojel®; Avebe, Foxhol, The Netherlands).
Cross-linked polyvinylpyrrolidone (PolyplasdoneXL®; GAF Corp., New York, USA).
Castor oil (USP XXI grade; C. Erba, Milano, Italy).
FD & C lake Yellow 6 (Eigenmann & Veronelli SpA, Milano, Italy).
Glycerol palmitostearate (Precirol AT05; Gattefossè, Saint Priest, France).

Preparation of ibuprofen granulate (granulate A)

830 g of ibuprofen and 170 g of corn starch were mixed (Erweka LK 5; Heusenstamm, FRG) and the resulting mixture was wetted with 200 ml of a 2.5% w/v methylcellulose aqueous solution. The wet mixture was forced through an 800 μm screen to obtain a granulate which, after partial drying at 40°C in an air-circulating oven, was forced through a 420 μm screen. The dried granulate was then mixed in a Turbula apparatus (type T2A; Basel, Switzerland) with corn starch (2%), sodium starch glycolate (2%), cross-linked polyvinylpyrrolidone (2%) and magnesium stearate (0.5%), to obtain granulate A.

Preparation of barrier granulate (granulate B)

150 g of Methocel K15M, 50 g of Methocel K4M, 400 g of mannitol, 280 g of talc and 10 g of Yellow 6 lake were kneaded with 200 ml of a 10% w/v polyvinylpyrrolidone alcoholic solution and the wet mass was forced through a 420 μm screen.

The granulate was dried at 40°C and then was mixed with magnesium stearate (1%), to obtain granulate B.

Preparation of the three-layer tablets

The tablets were prepared using a multilayer tablet press having three loading stations (Manesty layer press; Liverpool, UK) equipped with a punch set (13 mm diameter); the first and third loading stations were filled with granulate A, the second being filled with granulate B. The die filling was adjusted to fill 400 mg of the granulate A (equivalent to 300 mg of Ibuprofen) from stations 1 and 3 and 100 mg of granulate B from station 2. The compression force of the final tableting step was about 25 kN.

Operating as described, cylindrical three-layer tablets were prepared, weighing about 900 mg and having two layers of active substance separated by a barrier layer of water swellable polymer mixture (granulate B).

Film coating procedure

A nude three-layer tablet was placed in a specially designed rotating bored holder so that only one of the drug layers was lodged into the holder itself, one portion of the tablet being exposed.

The exposed surface of the tablet (barrier plus the second drug layer) was then coated by spraying a 5% w/v solution of ethylcellulose in 1:1 methyl alcohol:dichloromethane in order to obtain a film of thickness 0.20±0.05 mm.

In vitro *disintegration and release tests*

(1) A modified USP XXI disintegration test apparatus (4000 ml beaker instead of 1000 ml low-form beaker) was used to control the finished systems.
(2) the systems were tested in 4000 ml of pH 7.2 phosphate buffer, at 37°C.

The ibuprofen concentration was determined spectrophotometrically at 264 nm (SPECTRACOMP 602; Advanced Products, Milan, Italy). This procedure allowed us to determine by means of the same experiment

(i) the disintegration time of the immediate dose,
(ii) the dissolution rate of the immediate dose,
(iii) the resistance of both the barrier and the container,
(iv) the dissolution rate of the remaining dose.

In vivo *experiments*

A preliminary study involving two healthy adult volunteers was carried out. Each subject received a single oral administration of the following dosage forms:

(a) conventional marketed plain tablets (300 mg of Ibuprofen);
(b) Conventional plain tablets prepared with granulate A (300 mg of Ibuprofen); two preparations differing in particle size distribution of the active principle;

(c) pulsed release system (2×300 mg of Ibuprofen).

Collection of blood samples (10 ml) was effected over 12 h following dosing. Plasma was separated by centrifugation and stored at −20°C until analysed. ibuprofen concentration was determined by HPLC using the method described in ref. 14.

RESULTS AND DISCUSSION

Structural characteristics of the systems

The system prepared is presented in Fig. 1.

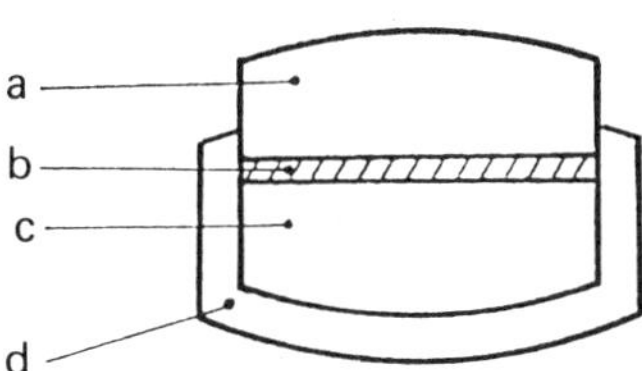

Fig. 1 — Schematic representation of the prepared pulsed release system: a, layer containing the immediately available dose of drug (first dose); b, barrier of swellable polymeric material; c, layer containing the second dose of drug; d impermeable film container.

In vitro testing

The system works as follows: on contact with the dissolution medium, the uncoated layer (a) rapidly disintegrates, leaving the remaining part of the system intact. The dissolution medium will then come into contact with the barrier (b), slowly interacting with it. The barrier delays the interaction between the dissolution medium and the second dose layer (c) for a time depending on its composition and thickness. As a result of medium–polymer interaction, the barrier slowly becomes viscous and its mechanical resistance decreases. When a sufficient amount of water crosses the barrier, the disintegrants present in layer c swell, thus developing a disintegrating force. The barrier breaks and the disintegration of the third layer containing the second dose of ibuprofen occurs.

The disintegrating force developed by the two doses of the drug on contact with aqueous fluids is the energy source for the delivery of active substance; it has been obtained using *superdisintegrants* (e.g. Polyplasdone XL®, Primojel®).

On *in vitro* testing when the pulsed release system is immersed in the dissolution medium, the following can be observed:

(a) rapid disintegration of the uncoated part of the system (<5 min), leading to a fast dissolution of the first dose;
(b) slow gelling of the barrier;
(c) disintegration and dissolution of the second dose of the drug on breaking of the barrier.

Figs 2 and 3 show the dissolution profiles of the first and second doses of the drug respectively.

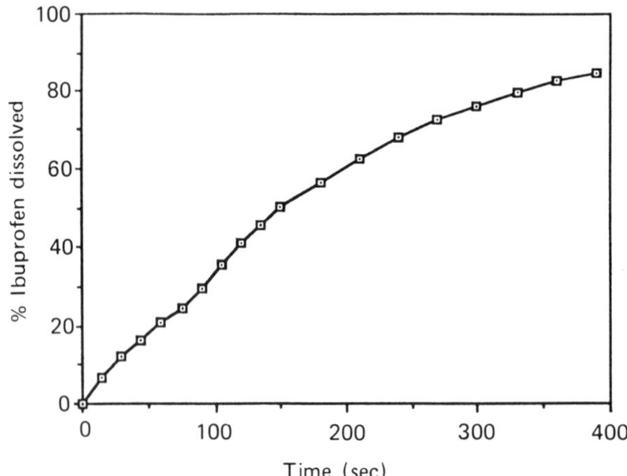

Fig. 2 — Dissolution profile of the first dose of ibuprofen (pH 7.2 phosphate buffer, 37°C, mean of six replicates).

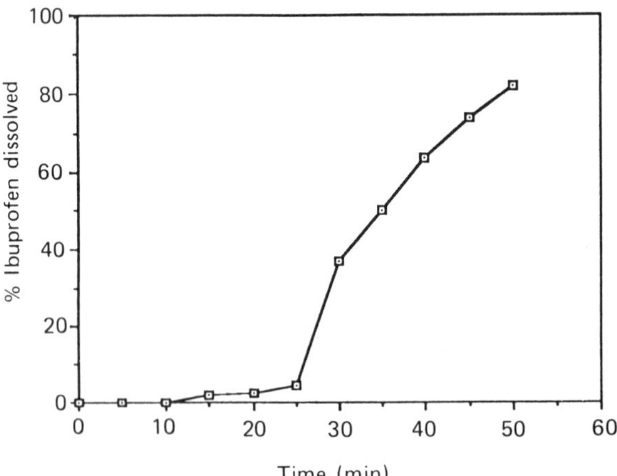

Fig. 3 — Dissolution profile of the second dose of ibuprofen (pH 7.2 phosphate buffer, 37°C, mean of six replicates).

The lag time evident in the dissolution profile of the second dose is determined by the progressive gelation of the intermediate barrier; in addition, since the dissolution medium permeates the barrier very slowly and wets the third layer, the disintegrant efficiency could be reduced, thus resulting in a significant decrease of drug dissolution rate.

In vivo **experiments**

Preliminary plasma levels obtained in a few subjects in order to verify the dependence of the *in vivo* pattern on the structure of the whole system and on the type, amount and characteristics of the drug and the polymers used are very promising.

Fig. 4 shows the plasma profiles obtained after oral administration of two plain tablets of 300 mg of ibuprofen prepared with two different batches of active principle, having differing particle size distributions (d_{vs}=11.5 μm and 5 μm), compared with a conventional marketed ibuprofen tablet.

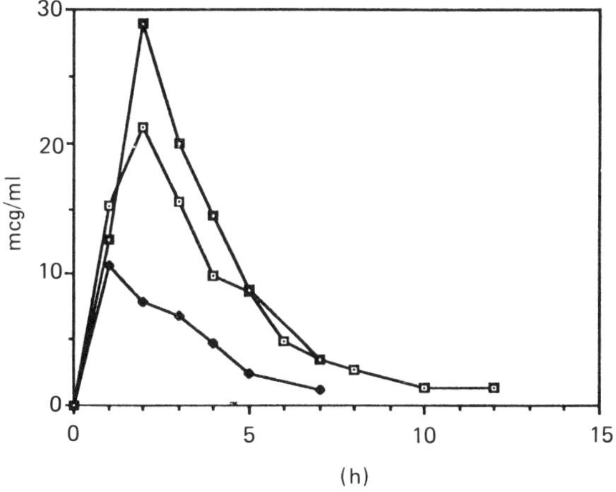

Fig. 4 — ibuprofen plasma levels following administration of the following: ⊡, ibuprofen 300 mg conventional marketed tablets; ■, ibuprofen (d_{vs}=11.5 μm) 300 mg conventional tablets; ■, ibuprofen (d_{vs}=5 μm) 300 mg conventional tablets. Each curve is the mean of the data from two subjects.

The plasma levels are strongly dependent on the specific surface area of the ibuprofen powder.

The differences in absorption rate and bioavailability between the tablets prepared with the differing batches of ibuprofen are clearly evident despite the fact that their *in vitro* dissolution profiles can be practically superimposed when tested according to the USP XXI *ibuprofen Tablets* monograph.

Fig. 5 shows an example of the plasma levels after administration of the pulsed release system to two volunteers. As can be seen from Fig. 5, in both cases there are two peaks. The first peak is 20 μg ml^{-1} after about 1 h, and the second is 16–20 μg ml^{-1} after 4.5–5 h; there is an evident delay in the absorption of the second

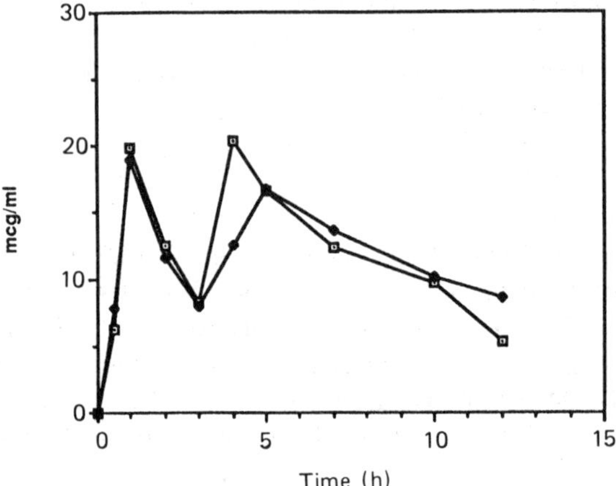

Fig. 5 — ibuprofen plasma levels following administration of pulsed release system to two subjects: ⊡, first subject; ■, second subject.

dose which appears to correlate quite well with the *in vitro* performance of the pulsed system.

CONCLUSIONS

The *in vitro* disintegration and dissolution tests of the pulsed system, obtained with a suitable blend of polymers and appropriate processing, are in good agreement with the *in vivo* blood levels and pattern.

Despite the problems posed by the pharmacokinetic and physicochemical characteristics of ibuprofen (small therapeutic window, erratic absorption owing to its poor solubility, etc.), this pulsed release system results in good separation of the two plasma peaks (indicating that there is in fact delayed release of the second drug dose) at the desired concentrations.

These preliminary results, which substantiate the initial hypothesis, show the system to be very promising.

ACKNOWLEDGEMENTS

This work was supported by a grant from FARMARESA (Research Contract 1986/87). The authors are grateful to Mrs. M. C. Sacchi for assistance in text and figure preparation.

REFERENCES

[1] U. Conte, P. Columbo, C. Caramella and A. La Manna, *Proc. Symp. on Polymers in Medicine,* Plenum, New York, 1983, p. 179.

[2] U. Conte, P. Colombo, C. Caramella, G. P. Bettinetti, F. Giodano and A. La Manna, *Farmaco, Ed. Prat.*, **39**, 67 (1984).
[3] P. Colombo, U. Conte, C. Caramella, A. Gazzaniga and A. La Manna, *J. Control. Release,* **1**, 283 (1985).
[4] A. La Manna, U. Conte, P. Colombo, A Gazzaniga, G. C. Santus and M. E. Sangalli, *Italian Patent Appl. 20708 A/86,* 28 May, 1986.
[5] A. Gazzaniga, U. Conte, P. Colombo, M. E. Sangalli, C. Caramella and A. La Manna, *Polymers in Medicine III,* Elsevier, Amsterdam, 1988, p. 201.
[6] A. Gazzaniga, M. E. Sangalli, U. Conte, C. Caramella, P. Colombo and A. La Manna, *Proc. Int. Symp. Control. Release Bioact. Mater.*, **15**, 464 (1988).
[7] P. Colombo, U. Conte, A. Gazzaniga, C. Caramella and A. La Manna, *Acta Pharm. Technol.*, **33**, 15 (1987).
[8] U. Conte, P. Colombo, A. Gazzaniga, M. E. Sangalli and A. La Manna, *Biomaterials,* **9**, 489 (1988).
[9] P. Colombo, U. Conte and A. La Manna, *Italian Patent Appl. 19772 A/85,* 31 May, 1985.
[10] P. Colombo, L. Maggi, A. Gazzaniga, U. Conte, A. La Manna and N. A. Peppas, *Proc. Int. Symp. Control. Release Bioact. Mater.*, **15**, 40 (1988).
[11] G. Leyendecker, T. Struve and E. J. Plotz, *Arch. Gynecol.*, **229**, 117 (1980).
[12] D. L. Wise, D. J. Trantolo, R. T. Marino and I. P. Kitchell, *Adv. Drug Delivery Rev.*, **1**, 19 (1987).
[13] P. Colombo, A. La Manna and U. Conte, *Italian Patent Appl. 19064 A/87,* 13 January, 1987.
[14] G. F. Lockwood and J. G. Wagner, *J. Chromatogr.*, **232**, 335 (1982).

8

Topical release and permeation studies of propranolol hydrochloride from hydrophilic polymeric matrices

C. Pillai, A. Baber and **F. M. Plakogiannis**
Division of Pharmaceutics and Industrial Pharmacy, Arnold & Marie Schwartz College of Pharmacy, Long Island University, Brooklyn, NY 11201, USA

SUMMARY

In vitro release of propranolol hydrochloride, a commonly used β-adrenergic blocking agent, form various hydrophilic polymeric gels was studied. These included: Methocel®, Avicel®, polyvinyl alcohol, methyl cellulose and gelatin-based systems. Several ingredients, such as ethyl alcohol, dimethylsulphoxide (DMSO) and polyethylene glycol 400 were included in the formulations at various concentration levels for possible enhancement of drug release. The release studies were carried out using a cellulose membrane and hairless mouse skin as the diffusion barriers. The general rank order for the drug release through these membranes was observed to be as follows: Methocel® matrix>Avicel® CL-611 matrix>PVA–gelatin matrix>emulsion base. The inclusion of other ingredients in the formulations had little or no effect in enhancing the drug release. However, when the hairless mouse skin was soaked in DMSO for 1 h prior to use in the diffusion studies, the drug release was increased by 40%. The amount of propranolol hydrochloride released from the Methocel® matrix in 24 h was observed to be well within the therapeutic range, i.e. 0.21–0.81 mg per litre.

The *in vitro* release data were treated with various kinetic models to assess the diffusion coefficient, the partition coefficient and the permeability coefficient. Using this information, the formulations evaluation were screened from their suitability to deliver propanolol hydrochloride as a topical dosage form.

INTRODUCTION

Propranolol, an effective β-adrenergic blocking agent, was first introduced on the market as Inderal® by Ayerst laboratories, Inc. [1,2]. It was approved by the Food and Drug Administration initially for the treatment of cardiac arrhythmias in 1968, then for the treatment of angina pectoris in 1973 and finally as an antihypertensive agent in 1976. In addition to its effectiveness in the management of hypertension [3–8], it has been found to be useful in the treatment of hyperthyroidism [9]. Lately it has been indicated in the prophylaxis of migraine headache.

Propranolol is chemically a naphthol derivative (*dl*-(isopropylamino)-3-(l-naphthyloxy)-2-propanol). It is a racemic mixture, and the laevo form is the active β-adrenergic blocking agent [10]. After oral administration, it is completely absorbed [11]. However, the systemic availability is relatively low with considerable variation in plasma levels [12,13]. The hepatic extraction of propranolol is about 80–90%, and thus the main route of drug elimination is via hepatic metabolism [14]. One of the major metabolites of propranolol is 4-hydroxypropranolol, and the half-life has been reported to be 3±1–1/2 h [15–18]. Since the drug is rapidly metabolized after oral administration, it necessitates a multiple dosage after oral strict patient compliance.

The therapeutically effective concentration of propranolol has been established to be 0.21–0.81 mg per litre and the lethal concentration in the range 8–12 mg per litre [19].

Some of untoward effects of propranolol therapy are associated with the gastrointestinal tract, i.e. nausea, vomiting, mild diarrhoea and constipation, etc. The drug also affects the central nervous system causing lassitude, asthenia, visual disturbances and rarely hallucination. It may sometimes produce erythmatous rash with fever, sore throat, orthostatic hypotension, hypoglycaemia and bronchospasm.

At present, the pharmaceutical industry has invested a major slice of its research and development efforts in the development of novel drug delivery dosage forms. Generally, this is to maximize the drug efficacy and to minimize the side effects usually associated with the conventional oral route of drug administration. In addition to the popular controlled release dosage forms, the transdermal route of drug delivery is being extensively investigated. Consequently, several transdermal patches of clinically important drugs, such as scopolamine and transglycerin, have been successfully marketed. These types of transdermal drug delivery systems are designed to deliver the medication gradually into the body in a preprogrammed fashion. These dosage forms present the drug to the patient in a most convenient and acceptable manner [20].

In the light of these observations and the newer trends in product formulation, it was decided to study the *in vitro* release and permeation of propranolol hydrochloride from various hydrophilic polymeric matrices using the cellulose membrane and the hairless mouse skin as the diffusion barriers and to evaluate the effects of some of the additive ingredients known to enhance drug release from dermatological bases.

EXPERIMENTAL

Materials

The materials used were propranolol hydrochloride (Ayerst Laboratories Inc., Rouses Point, NY), Methocel® K100M (Dow Chemical Corporation, MI), methyl paraben (Amend Drug and Chemical Co., NJ), propyl paraben (Amend Drug and Chemical Co., NJ), gelatin A-260 (Amend Drug and Chemical Co., NJ), glycerin (Amend Drug and Chemical Co., NJ), propylene glycol (Ruger Chemical Co. Inc., NJ), methyl cellulose (Ruger Chemical Co. Inc. NJ), Avicel® CL-611 (FMC Corporation Inc., IN), polyvinyl alcohol (Aldrich Chemical Co. Inc., WI), hydrophilic ointment base (Pharmoderm Inc., New York, NY), ethanol (95%; US Industrial Chemicals Co., NY), polyethylene glycol 400 (J. T. Baker, Chemical Co., NJ) and dimethyl sulphoxide (Fischer Scientific Company Inc. NJ).

Equipment

Franz diffusion cells apparatus (Crown & Glass Company Inc., NJ), constant temperature water bath (Yamato Scientific Co. Ltd., Japan) and spectrophotometer (Shimadzu Siesakusho Ltd, Japan) were used.

Preparation of samples

Matrix formulations

All ingredients of the individual formulation as shown in Table 1 were accurately weighed for the batch size. The polymer was slowly dispersed in a portion of previously heated water at 80±2°C and another portion of water at room temperature was added and mixed. Propranolol hydrochloride and other ingredients including additives were predissolved and then incorporated in the batch at 40±2°C. All samples prepared were then stored in glass containers.

Table 1 — Formulations

Ingredient	Amount (% w/w)			
	A[a]	B	C	D
Propranolol hydrochloride	1.00	1.00	1.00	1.00
Methocel® K100M	2.00	—	—	—
Avicel® CL-611	—	8.00	—	—
Methyl cellulose 400 cps	—	2.00	—	—
Polyvinyl alcohol (20%)	—	—	50.00	—
Gelatin A-260	—	—	10.00	—
Hydrophilic ointment	—	—	—	80.00
Glycerin	—	15.00	—	—
Propylene glycol	10.00	—	10.00	—
Methyl paraben	0.20	0.20	0.20	0.20
Propyl paraben	0.05	0.05	0.05	0.05
Additive(s)	q.s.	—	—	—
Purified water q.s.	100.00	100.00	100.00	100.00

[a] Formulation A was also made at 0.5%, 2% and 3% concentration of drug.

Emulsion base formulation
All ingredients of the emulsion base formulation (Table 1) were accurately weighed for the batch size. The drug and parabens premixed in water were then added to the previously melted emulsion base at 50±2°C and stirred until completely mixed. The samples prepared were cooled to room temperature and stored in glass containers.

Assay procedure for propranolol hydrochloride
Plots of absorbance vs. wavelength for solutions of propranolol hydrochloride in water and buffer pH 6, USP [21], were developed. The maximum absorbance values observed were 290 nm for water and buffer solutions of the drug. Beer's law was followed for 1–20 µg/ml concentrations. The stability of drug was determined in the buffer solution. After 24 h at 37°C no potency loss was noted.

Content uniformity
All samples prepared were analysed for propranolol hydrochloride content. Only samples with 100% ±10% drug contents were used in these studies.

IN VITRO DIFFUSION STUDIES

The *in vitro* diffusion studies for each sample were carried out by using the Franz diffusion cells with a diffusional area of about 1.76 cm^2. The acceptor compartment of the apparatus was filled with the buffer solution pH 6, USP [21], and maintained at 37±0.5°C via a circulating water system. The diffusion membrane (the cellulose membrane with a molecular weight cut-off point of 1000 or the hairless mouse skin) previously prepared was placed between the donor and the acceptor compartments of the assembly. An accurately weighed 4 g of sample was then placed in the donor cell and the diffusion process was started. The solution in the acceptor compartment was continuously stirred with a small magnetic stirrer to maintain the sink conditions. Aliquots from the receptor cells were removed at 0.5, 2, 4, 8 and 24 h time intervals and replaced with equal amounts of fresh buffer solution to maintain the diffusion volume. These solutions were then diluted appropriately with buffer solution and analysed spectrophotometrically.

Preparation of the hairless mouse skin
A set of three hairless mice about 6–8 weeks old were sacrificed for each experiment by snapping the spinal cord at the neck. The circular section of the abdominal portion of the skin was excised, sufficient to fit in the diffusion apparatus. The adhering fat and visceral debris were carefully removed from each sample of the skin and soaked in normal saline solution just prior to their use in the diffusion studies.

RESULTS AND DISCUSSION

Release–permeation studies using the cellulose membrane
In vitro release data of propranolol hydrochloride from the four formulations evaluated ovr a 24 h period are shown in Table 2. The decreasing rank order of drug

release from these samples was observed to be as follows: Methocel® matrix> Avicel® CL-611 matrix>PVA–gelatin matrix>emulsion base. The Methocel®

Table 2 — *In vitro* diffusion data from various formulations evaluated using the cellulose membrane

Sample	Drug release (mg±SD)/h)				
	0.5 h	2.0 h	4.0 h	8.0 h	24.0 h
Formulation A	1.30±0.09	2.55±0.08	3.85±0.12	5.90±0.04	11.75±0.11
Formulation B	0.45±0.00	1.30±0.09	2.10±0.15	3.15±0.15	7.20±0.15
Formulation C	0.46±0.06	1.35±0.08	2.48±0.12	4.08±0.12	6.53±0.00
Formulation D	0.21±0.07	0.46±0.07	0.92±0.14	1.38±0.22	2.42±0.14

Average of three determinations.

matrix, formulation A, exhibited the maximum release of the drug, whereas the drug released was at a minimum from the PVA–gelatin matrix, formulation C. This could be attributed to the possible cross-linkages formed between the two polymers which thus restricted the movement of the drug molecules within the gel. The release of propranolol hydrochloride from the emulsion base, formulation D, was relatively low compared with all the hydrophilic polymeric gel formulations. This suggests that, for a water-soluble drug such as propranolol hydrochloride, polymeric-gel-based formulations are clearly the better vehicles for developing such dosage forms.

To analyse the *in vitro* data in terms of more meaningful parameters, the data were first treated with a simplified Higuchi equation [22]:

$$Q = 2C_0(Dt/\pi)^{1/2} \qquad (1)$$

where Q is the amount of drug released per unit area $(\text{cm})^2$, C_0 is the initial quantity of the drug (mg), D is the diffusion coefficient, t is the time after application (h).

As the initial quantity of the drug (C_0), the diffusion coefficient (D) and π are essentially constants, equation (1) was reduced to

$$Q = K't^{1/2} \qquad (2)$$

The data were then treated with equation (2), and the cumulative amounts of drug released (Q) were plotted against the square root of the time ($t^{1/2}$) (Fig. 1). Excellent linearity was found, confirming that the release–permeation data followed the Higuchi model.

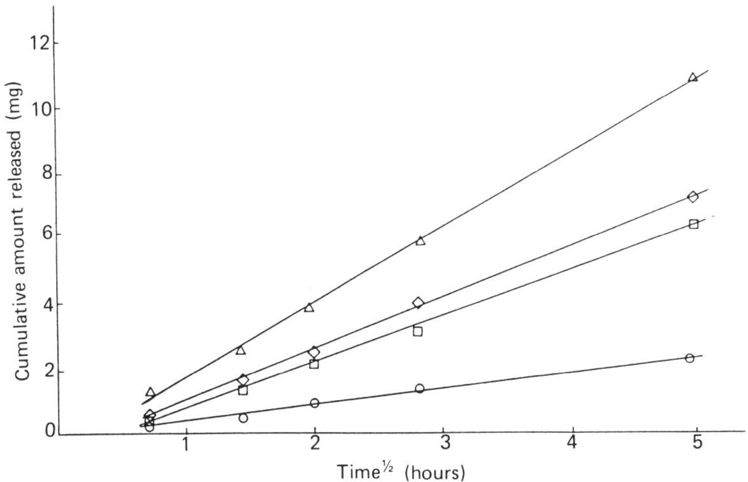

Fig. 1 — Diffusion profile of propranolol hydrochloride as a function of square root of time ($t^{1/2}$) from different polymeric matrices: △, Methocel® matrix; ◇, Avicel® CL-611 matrix; □, PVA–gelatin matrix; ○, emulsion base.

Since the Methocel® matrix, formulation A, gave the maximum drug release, several additives such as 95% ethanol, polyethylene glycol 400 and DMSO were added to it at 5%, 10% and 15% concentration levels. Almost all additives except for ethanol at the 5% level adversely affected the *in vitro* drug release (Table 3).

Furthermore, the effects of variations in polymer and drug concentration on the drug release from formulation A were evaluated. The polymer concentration was changed from 2.0% to 1.5% and 3.0% levels (Table 4). The change in the polymer concentration does not influence the release of the drug. However, the variation on drug concentration in formulation A, revealed that the propranolol hydrochloride release was directly proportional to the amount of the active drug present. This could be attributed to the enhanced thermodynamic activity of the drug molecules in the matrix system due to the higher concentration of the drug (Table 5 and Fig. 2).

Permeation studies using hairless mouse skin

The Methocel® matrix, formulation A, was further investigated using the hairless mouse skin as the diffusion barrier. Here the drug release was observed to be reduced significantly to 1.3 mg/(24 h) compared with 11.75 mg/(24 h) through the cellulose membrane. The formulation was further modified with the inclusion of

Table 3 — *In vitro* release–permeation of propranolol hydrochloride from Methocel® matrix formulation in the presence of the additive ingredients using cellulose membrane

Sample	Drug (%)	Amount released in 24 h (mg±SD)
Control		
Formulation A (Methocel® matrix)	1.0	11.75±0.11
With additives		
Ethanol		
5%	1.0	12.60±0.39
10%	1.0	10.75±0.31
15%	1.0	10.40±0.17
PEG-400		
5%	1.0	9.15±0.15
10%	1.0	7.05±0.03
15%	1.0	7.15±0.31
DMSO		
5%	1.0	10.65±0.30
10%	1.0	8.90±0.38
15%	1.0	7.75±0.46

Average of three determinations.

Table 4 — Drug release from Methocel® matrix formulation containing varied concentrations of polymer using the cellulose membrane

Time (h)	Drug released (mg±SD)		
	I	II	III
0.5	1.35±0.15	1.30±0.09	1.58±0.19
2.0	5.90±0.58	2.55±0.08	4.79±0.44
4.0	9.65±0.17	3.85±0.12	6.86±0.45
8.0	11.95±0.23	5.90±0.04	9.89±0.31
24.0	13.73±0.00	11.75±0.11	13.04±0.50

Average of three determinations.
I, drug:polymer ratio=1:1.5; II, drug:polymer ratio=1:2.0; III, drug:polymer ratio=1:3.0.

Table 5 — Drug release from Methocel® matrix formulation containing varied concentrations of propranolol hydrochloride

Drug (%)	Polymer (%)	Drug released in 24 h	
		(mg±SD)	(%)
0.5	2.0	4.85±0.16	24.25
1.0	2.0	11.75±0.11	29.38
2.0	2.0	16.85±0.38	21.06
3.0	2.0	33.33±0.34	27.78

Average of three determinations.

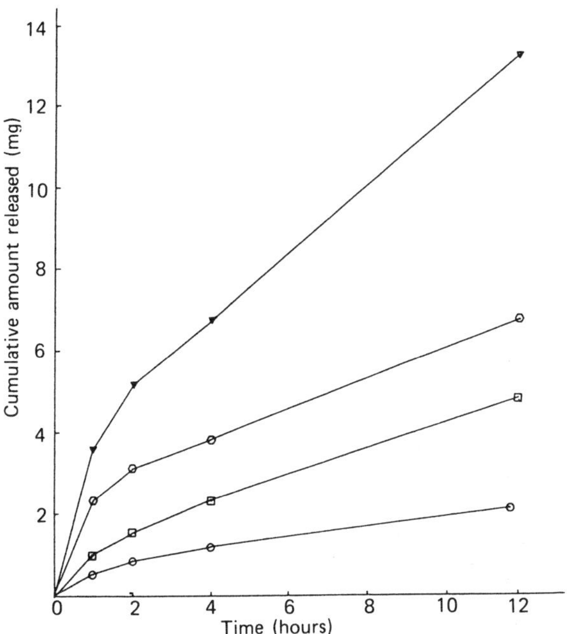

Fig. 2 — Effect of drug loading on the release profile of propranolol hydrochloride from Methocel® matrix: ▽, 3.0%; ⬡, 2.0%; □, 1.0%; ○, 0.5%.

DMSO in an effort to enhance drug release through the hairless mouse skin. When the diffusion membrane itself was soaked with DMSO for 1 h prior to its use, the drug release–permeation was increased by 40% (Table 6 and Fig. 3). The release patterns of the drug were linear from the samples containing in some way small amounts of DMSO. The sample without DMSO provided linear release only up to the first 12 h

Table 6 — Effect of DMSO on the permeability of propranolol hydrochloride from Methocel® matrix diffusion experiment through hairless mouse skin

I		II		III	
Time (h)	Concentration (mg±SD)	Time (h)	Concentration (mg±SD)	Time (h)	Concentration (mg±SD)
0	0	0	0	0	0
1	0.21±0.17	1	—	1	0.28±0.03
2	0.26±0.18	2	0.19±0.01	2	0.31±0.01
4	0.34±0.04	4	0.26±0.02	4	0.39±0.03
8	0.53±0.06	8	0.37±0.03	8	0.57±0.04
12	0.72±0.08	12	0.47±0.03	12	0.73±0.03
24	0.81±0.05	24	0.79±0.09	24	1.13±0.08

I, Methocel® matrix+skin; II, Methocel® matrix+5% DMSO skin; III, Methocel® matrix+skin (soaked in DMSO for 1 h).

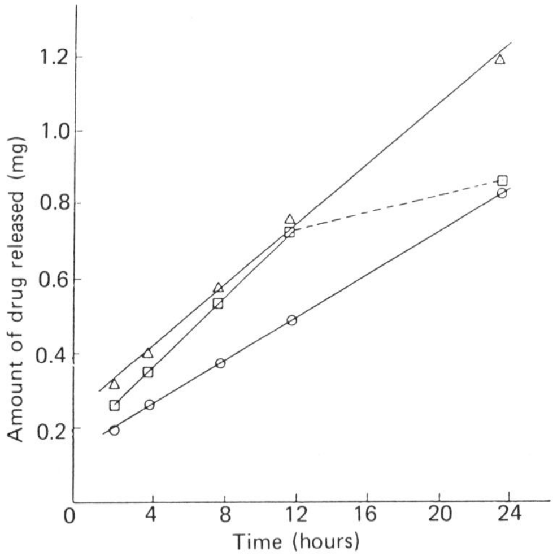

Fig. 3 — Diffusion profile of propranolol hydrochloride as a function of time (t) from Methocel® matrix through hairless mouse skin: □, matrix+skin; ○, matrix (5% DMSO)+skin; △, matrix+skin soaked in DMSO for 1 h.

period of the study. This could be attributed to the complicated processes involved in the passive diffusion of the drug through the skin. The linear release suggest that the drug release was zero order.

Using these data, some of the related parameters, i.e. rate constant (K), correlation coefficient (r) and the values for the Y intercepts, were calculated (Table 7). Comparing these data statistically, analyses were performed using the F test

Table 7 — Computed parameters for Methocel® matrix diffusion data through hairless mouse skin (up to 12 h)

Experiments	Correlation coefficient (r)	Rate constant (k) ($mg\,h^{-1}$)	Intercept (Y)
I Methocel® matrix+skin	0.9996	0.0463	0.1611
II Methocel® matrix+DMSO 5%+skin	0.9981	0.0277	0.1423
III Methocel® matrix+skin soaked in DMSO for 1 h	0.9996	0.0423	0.2245

(confidence interval, 95%). The drug release (Table 8) is significantly different when the hairless mouse skin was soaked in DMSO for 1 h compared with that from the Methocel® matrix formulation containing DMSO at the 5% level.

Table 8 — Permeability rate of propranolol hydrochloride from Methocel® matrix diffusion study through hairless mouse skin (comparative data)

Experiments	Permeability rate		Statistical significance[b]
	Concentration[a] (mg±SD)	(%)	
I Methocel® matrix+skin	0.81±0.05	2.02	—
II Methocel® matrix+skin+5% DMSO	0.79±0.09	1.98	NS
III Methocel® matrix+skin soaked in DMSO for 1 h	1.13±0.08	2.83	SS

[a] Concentration represents average of three determinations.
[b] Statistical analysis performed by the F test and confidence interval (95%) methods: NS, statistically not significant; SS, statistically significant.

The release data from various formulations using the cellulose membrane as the diffusion barrier were used to calculate the values for the diffusion coefficient (D), the permeability coefficient (P) and the partition coefficient (P_c) (Table 9). From

Table 9 — Computed values of permeability, diffusion and partition coefficients for different formulations

Formulations	Diffusion coefficient (D) ($\times 10^{-7}$ cm^2/s)	Permeability coefficient (P) ($\times 10^{-7}$ cm^2/s)	Partition coefficient (P_c) ($\times 10^{-1}$ cm^2/s)
Methocel® matrix	3.00	1.90	0.38
Avicel® CL-611 matrix	0.94	1.20	0.76
PVA–gelatin matrix	0.73	1.10	0.85
Emulsion base	0.11	0.40	2.30

this, it is observed that the sample with maximum drug release (Methocel® matrix formulation) has the highest diffusion coefficient value (3.0×10^{-7} cm^2/s), compared with the emulsion base formulation with only 0.11×10^{-7} cm^2/s. In addition, the highest permeability coefficient of 1.90×10^{-7} cm^2/s was obtained for this formulation, compared with the emulsion-based sample with a value of 0.40×10^{-7} cm^2/s. However, the partition coefficient is observed to be the lowest for the Methocel® matrix formulation (0.38×10^{-1} cm^2/s) compared with the value of 2.30×10^{-1} cm^2/s obtained with the emulsion base formulation, which gave the minimum release of the drug. For higher drug release the formulation should possess relatively high permeability and diffusion coefficient.

REFERENCES

[1] J. W. Black, A. F. Crowther, R. G. Shanks, I. H. Smith and A. C. Dornhost, *Lancet*, **1**, 1080 (1964).
[2] J. W. Black, W. M. Duncan and R. G. Shanks, *Br. J. Pharmacol.*, **25**, 577 (1965).
[3] B. N. C. Prichard, *Br. Med. J.*, **2**, 725 (1964).
[4] B. N. C. Prichard, *Br. Med. J.*, **1**, 1227 (1964).
[5] F. A. Richards, *Am. J. Cardiol.*, **18**, 384 (1966).
[6] B. N. C. Prichard and P. N. S. Gillman, *Am. J. Cardiol.*, **18**, 387 (1966).
[7] J. W. Paterson and C. T. Dollery, *Lancet*, **2**, 1148 (1966).
[8] H. J. Wall, *Clin. Pharmacol. Ther.*, **7**, 588 (1966).
[9] S. C. Harvey, *Remington's Pharmaceutical Sciences*, Mack, PA, 15th edn., 1975, p. 835.
[10] A. Goth, *Medical Pharamacology*, Mosby, St., Louis, MO, 10th ed., 1981, p. 206.
[11] J. W. Paterson, M. E. Conolly, C. T. Dollery, A. Heyes and R. G. Cooper, *Clin. Pharmacol.*, **2**, 127 (1970).
[12] A. Hussain, *J. Pharm. Sci.*, **69** (10), 1240 (1980).

[13] D. G. Shand, E. M. Nuckolls and J. A. Oates, *Clin. Pharmacol. Ther.*, **11**, 112 (1970).
[14] D. G. Shand, G. H. Evansand and A. S. Weiss, *Life Sci.*, **10**, (1), 1418.
[15] D. G. Shand, R. E. Rango, *Pharmacology*, **7**, 159 (1972).
[16] C. A. Chidsey, P. Morselli, G. Binachetti, A. Morganti, G. Laonetti and A. Zanchetti, *Circulation*, **52**, 313 (1975).
[17] R. Gomeni, G. Biachettie, R. Sega and P. L. Morselli, *J. Biopharm. Pharmacokinet.*, **5**, 183 (1977).
[18] O. B. Holland and N. M. Kaplan, *N. Engl. J. Med.*, **294**, 930 (1976).
[19] C. L. Winsk, *Clin. Chem.*, **22**, 832 (1976).
[20] F. Yates, H. Benson, R. Buckles, J. Urquhart and A. Zaffaroni, *Adv. Biomed. Eng.*, **5** (1975).
[21] *The United States Pharmacopia and National Formulary*, XXI, NF XVI, 1985, p. 1420.
[22] T. Higuchi, *J. Pharm. Sci.*, **50**, 874 (1961).

Multiparticulates

9

Polyacrylate (Eudragit retard) microspheres for oral controlled release of nifedipine: Formulation design and process optimization

A. Barkai, Y. V. Pathak and **S. Benita**†
Department of Pharmacy, School of Pharmacy, The Hebrew University of Jerusalem, PO Box 12065, Jerusalem 91120, Israel

SUMMARY

Nifedipine was incorporated in polyacrylate–polymethylcrylate microspheres using the solvent evaporation process. Optimal experimental conditions were found for the production of large batches of nifedipine microspheres based on Eudragit polymers. It was noted that the microspheres were not quite spherical and some of them, especially the large microspheres, collapsed and lost their spherical shape as a result of the existence of internal void volume as evidenced by scanning electron microscopy (SEM) examination of fractured nifedipine microspheres. It appeared that the experimental conditions used in the present study favoured the formation of microspheres of a new type. They could be defined as 'film-type' microspheres which consisted of spherical micromatrices comprising an internal void space and a polymeric membrane of variable thickness where the nifedipine was dispersed in either a molecular or a solid state depending on the payload. This was confirmed by differential scanning calorimetry analysis and SEM which detected drug crystals embedded on the microsphere surfaces at high drug content.

INTRODUCTION

Polyacrylate–polymethacrylate copolymers (Eudragits) are widely used as tablet adjuvants and coating polymers [1]. These polyacrylate polymers were also used for

† Author to whom correspondence should be addressed.

the microencapsulation of paracetamol, indomethacin and theophylline by means of a coacervation method involving phase separation from chloroform by a non-solvent addition technique [2,3]. Eudragit polymers have also recently received increased attention as microsphere wall materials [4–8].

Nifepidine, a systemic calcium channel blocking agent, practically insoluble in water and light sensitive, was selected since the drug exhibits all the required pharmacokinetic and physicochemical properties which make it a good candidate to be incorporated in a controlled release dosage form. Therefore, nifedipine has been incorporated in microspheres of Eudragit RS and RL. The polyacrylate microspheres were prepared using the solvent evaporation technique previously reported [4]. Production variables have been tested for the purpose of defining conditions for the design and production of large batches of these microspheres.

MATERIALS AND METHODS

Nifedipine conformed to USP XXI; Eudragit RS and RL were kindly provided by Roehm Pharma GmbH (Darmstadt, FRG); polyvinyl alcohol (PVA), MW of 14 000, was supplied by BDH Laboratory (Poole, UK).

Preparation of nifedipine microspheres on a small scale (2.5 g per batch of microspheres)

The preparation method previously reported was used [4]. Various amounts of nifedipine (50–1200 mg) were incorporated into a 2 g mixture of Eudragit RS and RL (1:1).

Method of preparation of large batches of nifedipine microspheres

After preparing a large number of batches in preliminary studies, the following optimal experimental conditions were finalized for the production of nifedipine microspheres. Water (1 l) containing 0.8% PVA was placed on a 3 l glass beaker. A solution comprising 25 g of Eudragit RS:RL (1:1) and nifedipine (1.25–12.5 g) in a known amount of methylene chloride (60–100 ml) was added to the aqueous phase through a separating funnel (4 cm diameter). The mixture was stirred at a constant rate by a Heidolph stirrer fitted with a digital counter and a four-blade impeller having a diameter of 15 cm. The agitation rate was varied from 200 to 750 rev/min. The resulting emulsion was agitated at room temperature for 16 h during which time the methylene chloride was evaporated. The solid microspheres were allowed to settle and the aqueous phase that contained the polymeric dispersing agent was replaced by distilled water using at least five washing and decantation steps. The microspheres were isolated by filtration, washed, eventually sieved (20 mesh) and dried overnight at 37°C. It should be emphasized that the entire manufacturing process was protected as much as possible from light. Duplicate batches were prepared for reproducibility evaluation. The following preparation parameters were varied: the volume of the organic solvent phase, rate of agitation and nifedipine concentration. Empty Eudragit microspheres were prepared using identical experimental conditions but in the absence of nifedipine.

Microsphere evaluation

Nifedipine content

Known amounts of nifedipine microspheres (20–100 mg) were dissolved in 50–100 ml of chloroform (analytical grade). Nifedipine was then assayed spectrophotometrically using a calibration curve at 338 nm. The dissolved Eudragit polymers did not absorb at this wavelength. Actual or measured drug contents were usually lower than the theoretical values owing to drug loss or partition to the aqueous phase during methylene chloride evaporation.

Microscopy studies

Optical microscopy and scanning electron microscopy (SEM) were used to evaluate the drug incorporation and surface shape of the microspheres prepared under the various conditions. Particle size was determined using a Tiyoda microscope. Samples of microspheres (180–200) were dispersed on a slide and their diameter was then sized using suitable objectives.

Determination of methylene chloride traces

The assay was carried out using a Varian gas chromatograph (model 5000 LC) under the following experimental condition. The oven injector and flame ionization detector temperatures were 125°C and 225°C respectively. A Porapak column was used, the eluent was N_2 at a flow rate of 30 ml/min and the injected volume 2 μl. Various concentrations of purified methylene chloride in purified methanol were injected (both solvents were distilled to discard any impurity which might interfere with the sensitive assay). Calibration curves were linear in the range 50–500 ppm (the limit of detection was 10 ppm). Methylene chloride detection in the microspheres was performed by dissolving various amounts (20–200 mg) of microspheres in 220 ml of purified methanol prior to the injection.

Differential scanning calorimetry

Differential thermal analysis (heating cycles of 90–200°C) of the pure nifedipine, empty Eudragit microspheres and microspheres containing various amounts of nifedipine was carried out to evaluate the internal structure after drug incorporation. This was achieved by means of a Mettler TA 3000 system.

The microspheres were also evaluated for their release kinetic profiles and stability at three temperatures.

RESULTS AND DISCUSSION

In the process of batch upgrading two main technical problems were identified based on research experience gained during previous work:

(a) the agitation system and equipment selection;
(b) the period of time at which methylene chloride should evaporate.

The approach used to resolve the various technical problems was based on the decision that the minimal amount of microspheres prepared per batch would be 25 g.

The agitation system and equipment selection

It was previously shown that the formation of a stable emulsion of methylene chloride in water was vital for the successful formation of individual microspheres [4,9]. Two main factors played an important role in the emulsification of methylene chloride in water and influenced the microsphere size: the interfacial tension of the methylene chloride droplets in the surrounding aqueous phase and the forces of shear within the fluid mass. The former tends to resist the distortion of droplet shape necessary for fragmentation into smaller droplets whereas the latter forces act to distort and ultimately to disrupt the droplets. The relationship between these forces largely determines the final size distribution of the methylene chloride in water emulsion which in turn controls the final size distribution of the solid microspheres formed.

Finally, the stirring system previously described was selected and was able to agitate efficiently 1 l of PVA aqueous solution producing an axial flow accompanied by marked turbulence in the immediate vicinity of the impeller.

The methylene chloride evaporation process

In the preparation of small batches, methylene chloride was allowed to evaporate at room temperature. The entire process lasted for 75–90 min [4]. In the present study, the minimum volume of methylene chloride required to dissolve 25 g of Eudragit mixture (RS:RL; 1:1) was 60 ml. This volume was dispersed in 1 l of aqueous phase. However, because of the high viscosity of the organic solution, it was very difficult to evaporate the methylene chloride within a few hours of mixing. Therefore, the emulsification temperature was raised to 40°C to effect methylene chloride evaporation in 3 h. The increase in temperature affected the microspheres which were accompanied by a significant amount of Eudragit debris instead of spherical microspheres. This could be attributed to the alteration of the protective effect of PVA which was probably sensitive to temperature variations. It was clear that microsphere formation should occur at room temperature. The use of optimal and efficient stirring conditions allowed for the evaporation of methylene chloride at room temperature, but more than 16 h were required to remove the organic solvent.

PVA acted as a protective polymer by being absorbed at the oil–water interface of the droplets to produce a steric barrier which prevented the coalescence of the droplets. Therefore PVA formed a stable emulsion of methylene chloride in water, even when nifedipine was dissolved in the methylene chloride phase. However, nifedipine tended to crystallize spontaneously in the aqueous phase of the emulsion or on the surface of the microspheres when solvent evaporation approached completion. This nifedipine crystal formation was detected even at a low drug payload of 5% (Fig. 1). Most of the free drug crystals that formed either floated in the water phase or were so loosely attached to the microspheres that they washed off during the isolation step. The loss of free drug crystals reduced the amount of nifedipine incorporated in the microspheres. Measured drug contents were always relatively high. Large amounts of nifedipine were not partitioned from the methylene chloride phase into the aqueous phase during the long fabrication process. This would account for the reduction in loss rate with increasing initial concentration of nifedipine as observed.

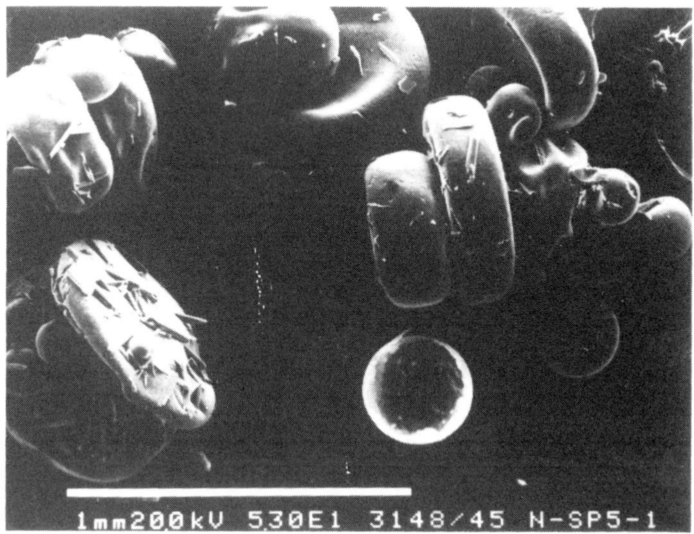

Fig. 1 — Scanning electron micrograph of nifedipine-loaded microspheres (4.7% w/w) prepared using 1 l of 0.8% polyvinyl alcohol solution, 25 g Eufragit RS:RL mixture. (1:1) in 80 ml methylene chloride stirred at 400 rev/min.

Methylene chloride residues in the microspheres

Nifedipine microspheres having a payload of either 4.6% or 31% (w/w) were stored at 4, 20 and 37°C and were examined for methylene chloride residue. No methylene chloride peak could be detected (10 ppm limit of detection) following dissolution in purified methanol and injection of 2 µl in the gas chromatograph. Identical results were obtained for the microspheres stored at various temperatures, indicating that effective removal of volatile solvent occurred following the separation and isolation process and before microsphere storage. From these results it can be concluded that less than 0.1% (v/w) methylene chloride is present in the solid microspheres calculated on the dried basis.

Differential scanning calorimetry analysis

This analytical method characterizes the nature of the drug encapsulated in the microspheres. There was no thermal event during the examination of empty microspheres. However, in the case of the melting phase transition of pure nifedipine, a sharp endotherm was observed at 172–173°C, corresponding exactly to the melting point of nifedipine (Fig. 2(a)) whereas no thermal event at all was detected in the microspheres containing 4.7% (w/w) nifedipine (Fig. 2(b)). The thermal behaviour of these nifedipine microspheres was similar to that observed with empty Eudragit microspheres.

It can therefore be deduced that nifedipine at this concentration in the Eudragit microspheres was present in either a molecular dispersion or a solid solution state. This was also confirmed by the SEM analysis. It can be seen from Figs 1 and 3 that

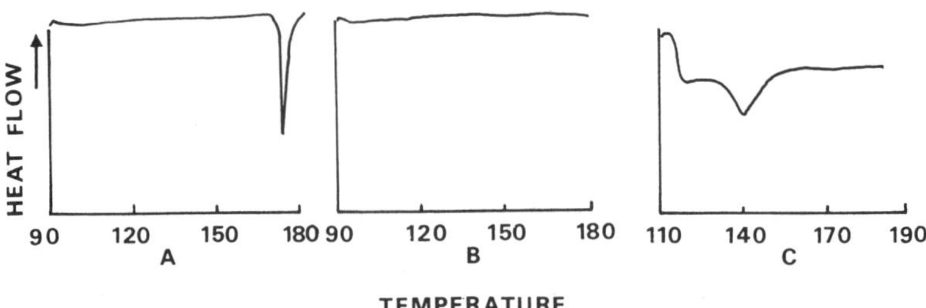

Fig. 2 — Differential thermal calorimetry analysis of (a) pure nifedipine and Eudragit microspheres containing (b) 4.7% nifedipine (c) 31% nifedipine.

microspheres containing up to 5% nifedipine had very smooth surfaces. There was no evidence of macroscopic pores. Formation of fine nifedipine crystals seemed to have no effect on the surface structure of the nifedipine microspheres when the drug payload was 4.8% (w/w). However, three microspheres did not appear totally spherical.

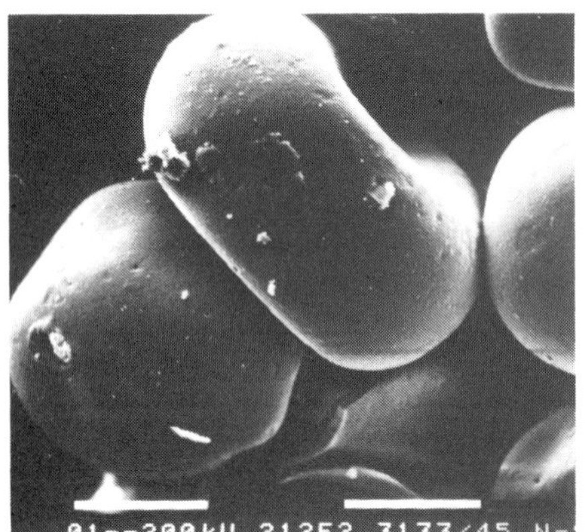

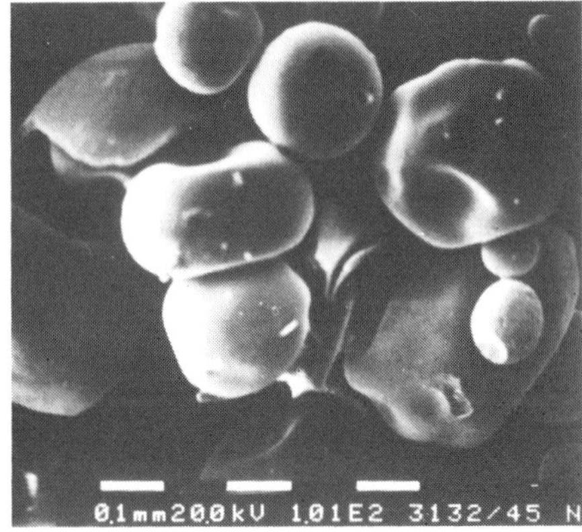

Fig. 3 — Scanning electron micrograph of well-washed nifedipine-loaded microspheres (4.7% w/w) at various magnifications. For experimental conditions see Fig. 1.

The nifedipine-loaded microspheres with a drug payload of 31% had a clear inflection of 139.6°C which could be attributed to the presence of crystalline domains in the microspheres (Fig. 2(c)). This peak was not close to the melting point of pure nifedipine, indicating that, during the methylene chloride evaporation phase, no recrystallization of pure nifedipine occurred within the microspheres, probably as a result of molecular interactions between nifedipine and the Eudragit polymers. Nevertheless, this inflection provided evidence that at least some of the nifedipine existed in the microsphere in a solid state. This evidence is consistent with the SEM examinations, which indicated that drug crystals were embedded on the microsphere surfaces (Fig. 4). It could be noted from Fig. 4 that the microspheres where not quite

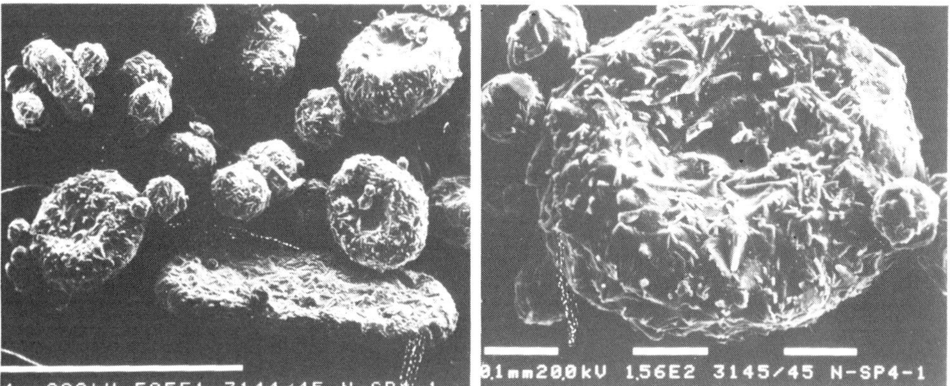

Fig. 4 — Scanning electron micrograph of nifedipine-loaded microspheres (31% w/w) at various magnifications. For experimental conditions, see Fig. 1.

spherical and some of them, especially the large microspheres, collapsed and lost their spherical shape owing to the existence of an internal void volume as evidenced by Fig. 5, exhibiting the internal structure of a fractured nifedipine microsphere

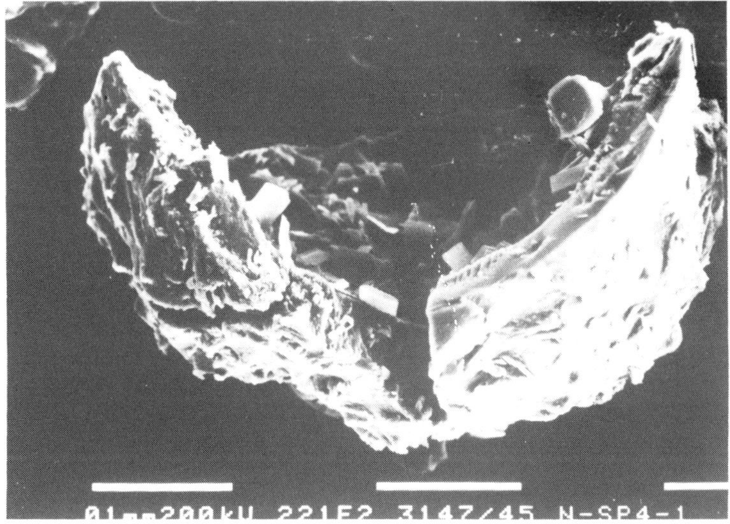

Fig. 5 — Scanning electron micrograph of a fractured nifedipine-loaded microsphere (31% w/w).

having a payload of 31%. This morphological depression could be attributed to the method used to prepare the microspheres for SEM evaluation. To visualize the microsphere, in SEM, a gold coating is imparted. During the gold coating process, the nifedipine microspheres which may have internal void volumes probably become deflated by the vacua required to carry out the coating process and account for the various wall collapses detected by SEM. Nevertheless, rehydration of the microspheres regenerated their spherical shape, as observed by means of an optical microscope. It is interesting to note that a microsphere preparation method based on a solvent evaporation process did not produce dense micromatrices as previously reported [4]. It should be emphasized that, when the nifedipine microspheres were prepared using identical experimental conditions but on a small laboratory scale with the total microsphere amount per batch not exceeding 2.5 g, dense, homogeneous, spherical micromatrices with the nifedipine either molecularly dispersed or dissolved in the polymer were obtained in (Fig. 6). Larger batches have therefore led to the

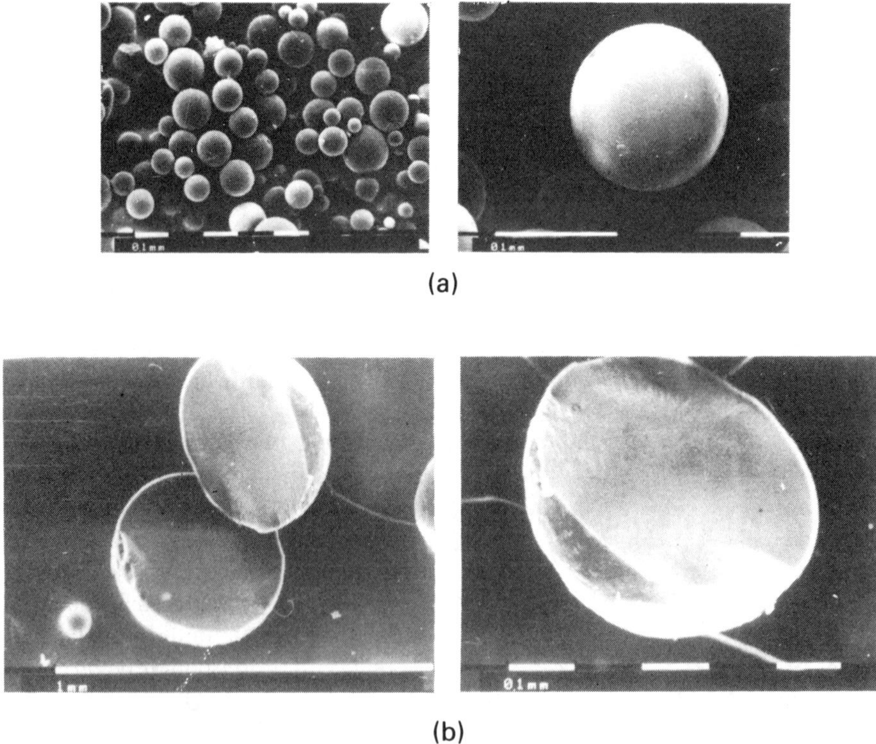

Fig. 6 — (a) Scanning electron micrograph of nifedipine-loaded microspheres (5% w/w) and (b) cross-sectional view of nifedipine-loaded microspheres (17% w/w) prepared on a small laboratory scale with the total microsphere amount per batch not exceeding 2.5 g.

formation of nifedipine-loaded microspheres with different morphological properties. However, in no case could these microspheres be defined as microcapsules, since there is no distinct core material (nifedipine) which is enclosed in the membranic envelope.

Effect of methylene chloride phase viscosity

The viscosity of the emulsified organic solvent phase was increased by reducing the volume of methylene chloride needed to dissolve 25 g of Eudragit mixture and 2.5 g of nifedipine. it could be seen from the results reported in Table 1 that the interbatch

Table 1 — Effect of initial methylene chloride viscosity on the nifedipine microsphere content

Methylene chloride phase volume (ml)	Measured drug content (%)		Drug loss (%)[a]	
	Batch 1	Batch 2	Batch 1	Batch 2
60	8.7	7.1	4.4	22
70	8.4	7.0	7.7	23
80	8.5	7.9	6.6	13.2
100	7.7	7.2	13.4	19

All the Eudragit microspheres (RS:RL; 1:1) had a theoretical content of 9.1% w/w nifedipine and were made by the evaporation process with 0.8% polyvinyl alcohol as the emulsifier at 600 rev/min.
[a][(theoretical drug content−measured drug content)/theoretical drug content]×100.

reproducibility was affected by the variation of the initial organic phase viscosity although no marked difference in measured drug payloads was observed with lower organic phase viscosities. Particle size analysis of microsphere batches prepared with different volumes of methylene chloride revealed a moderate increase in particle size with decreasing methylene chloride phase volume from 100 to 70 ml (Fig. 7). However, no marked difference could be observed between the populations of microspheres prepared using either 70 or 60 ml of methylene chloride. Nevertheless, there was a clear tendency for the mean measured diameter of the microspheres to increase with decreasing methylene chloride phase volume (289±119, 383±183, 432±134 and 450±175 μm for methylene chloride phase volumes of 100, 80, 70 and 60 ml respectively). The increase in particles size could be attributed to the increase in the methylene chloride phase viscosity caused by the diminution of the solvent volume which yielded larger emulsified droplets and consequently larger solid microspheres.

EFFECT OF STIRRING RATE

As expected, increasing the stirring rate decreased the mean diameter of the microspheres (Table 2) and the range of particle sizes obtained is close to the range

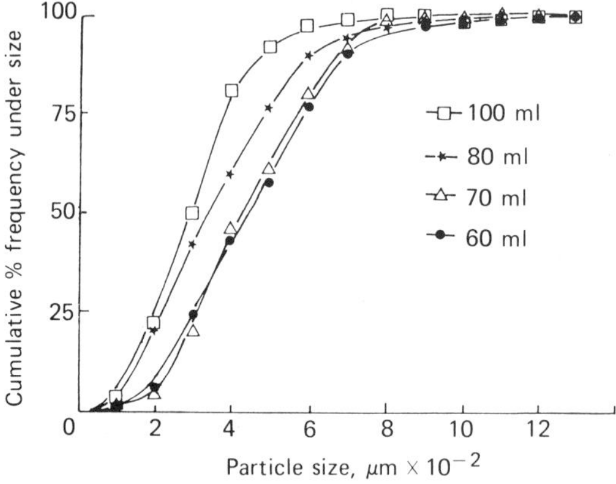

Fig. 7 — Cumulative frequency plot of nifedipine–Eudragit microspheres as a function of methylene chloride solution viscosity.

Table 2 — Effect of stirring rate on nifedipine microsphere content and size

Stirring rate (rev/min)	Meassured drug content (%)		Drug loss (%)[a]		Mean particle size (μm±SD)	
	Batch 1	Batch 2	Batch 1	Batch 2	Batch 1	Batch 2
200	6.8	6.5	25.3	28.6	567±302	780±304[b]
400	6.8	7.9	25.3	13.2	436±203	463±145
600	8.5	7.9	6.6	13.2	383±183	386±104
750	8.6	8.2	5.5	9.9	307±107	305±151

All Eudragit microspheres (RS:RL; 1:1) had a theoretical content of 9.1% w/w nifedipine and were prepared using 25 g of Eudragit mixture and 2.5 g of nifedipine dissolved in 80 ml initial methylene chloride volume phase.

[a]As in table 1.

[b]A large propoortion of the microspheres were elongated.

required for a multiparticulate dosage form. The width of the size distribution (SD) did not exhibit any tendency to vary with increasing stirring rate. Nevertheless, sieving could be performed in cases where a narrow range of microspheres is needed.

It also appears that stirring rate might affect the drug incorporation efficiency in the microspheres since less drug loss was observed with increasing agitation rate (Table 2). With regard to batch reproducibility, in either drug content or mean particle size, no marked difference was observed between the two batches prepared under identical experimental conditions, although some discrepancy was noted in the drug payload of the microspheres prepared using a stirring rate of 400 rev/min.

Effect of initial drug concentration

In an attempt to increase the nifedipine content of the microspheres, a number of experiments with increasing amounts of nifedipine were performed (Table 3). High

Table 3 — Effect of initial nifedipine concentration on microsphere drug content[a]

Initial nifedipine concentration (% w/w)	Measured drug content (%)[b]	Drug loss (%)[c]
4.8	4.6	3.5
9.1	7.4	19.2
16.6	14.3	14.0
23.0	18.8	18.4
33.3	31.1	6.6

[a]Microspheres were prepared using 1 l of 0.8% ppolyvinyl alcohol solution and 25 g Eudragit RSS:RL mixture (1:1) in 80 ml of methylene chloride stirred at 400 rev/min.
[b]Mean values of duplicates.
[c]As in Table 1.

payloads were achieved indicating that no rejection of nifedipine due to molecular interactions with the Eudragit polymers occurred. Drug loss values fluctuated with initial nifedipine concentration variation (Table 3).

It was also observed that increasing the nifedipine content in the microsphere altered the morphology of the microspheres (Figs 3 and 4). Clear findings were noted in the extreme cases, i.e. drug payloads of 4–8% or 31% w/w, but no clear conclusion could be drawn from the SEM observations of nifedipine microspheres having payloads of 10% to 25% w/w (Fig. 8). In contrast to the low-nifedipine-loaded microspheres (4.8% w/w), which exhibited smooth surfaces, in these intermediate paybloads formation of free nifedipine crystals probably affected the surface structure of the nifedipine microsphere which showed rippled and rough surfaces (Fig. 8). Also, nifedipine crystals were observed not to be attached firmly to the surface structure of the nifedipine microspheres. This phenomenon could be attributed to possible molecular interactions between the coating polymer and the nifedipine in that an excess of incorporated drug might result in recrystallization of nifedipine within the microspheres. This was further supported by the lack of any thermal event during the differential scanning calorimetry analysis of these microspheres.

Incorporation of increasing amounts of nifedipine within the microspheres gradually augmented their mean diameter and particle size distribution (Fig. 9). It could be observed that, in spite of a large degree of overlap in the particle size of the microspheres prepared using either the low or the high initial drug concentration, there was a clear tendency towards particle size increase with increasing nifedipine concentration. A similar behaviour was noted in the corresponding calculated mean diameters: 397±92, and 386±104 μm for microspheres with drug contents of 4.8%

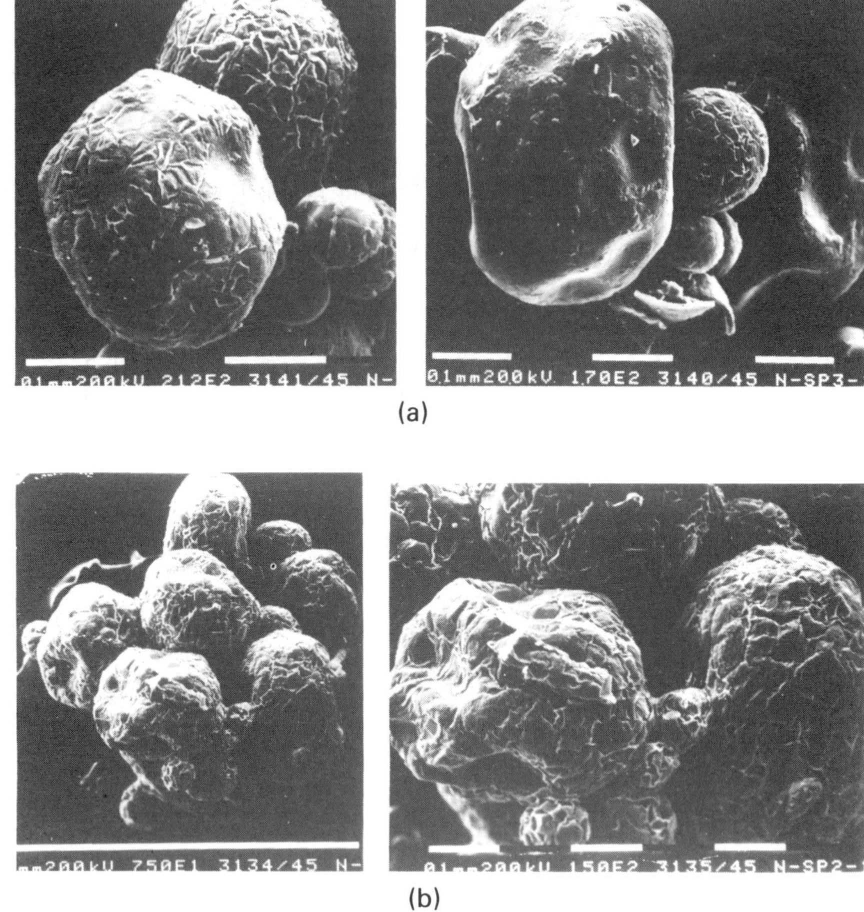

Fig. 8 — Scanning electron micrograph of Eudragit microspheres containing (a) 14.3% nifedipine and (b) 18.8% nifedipine at various magnifications. For experimental conditions see Fig. 1.

and 9.1% respectively, and 546±201 and 599±183 μm for nifedipine-loaded microspheres having payloads of 16.6% and 31% (w/w) respectively.

CONCLUSION

It appeared that the experimental conditions used in the present study favoured the formation of microspheres of a new type which could be defined as 'film-type' microspheres. They consisted of spherical micromatrices comprising an internal void space and a polymeric membrane of variable thickness where the drug is dispersed in either a molecular or a solid state depending on the payload.

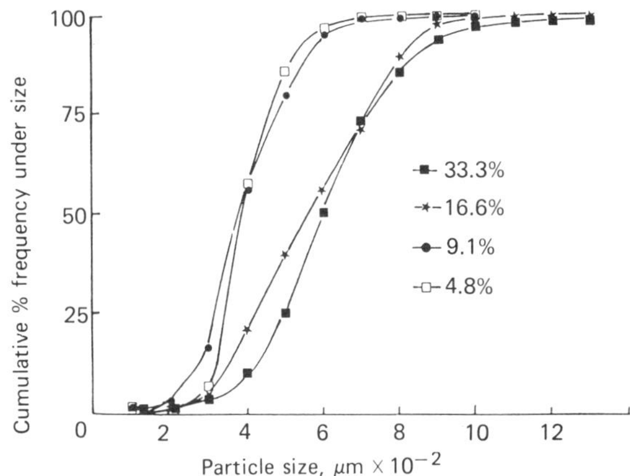

Fig. 9 — Cumulative frequency plot of nifedipine–Eudragit microspheres as a function of the initial nifedipine concentration. Microspheres were prepared using 1 l of 0.8% PVA and 25 g of Eudragit RS:RL mixture (1:1) in 80 ml of methylene chloride stirred at 400 rev/min.

ACKNOWLEDGEMENT

The authors would like to acknowledge the support given by Roehm Pharma, Darmstsadt, FRG.

REFERENCES

[1] K. O. R. Lehman and D. K. Dreher, *Pharm. Technol.*, **3**, 5 (1979).
[2] S. Benita, A. Hoffman and M. Donbrow, *J. Pharm. Pharmacol.*, **37**, 391 (1985).
[3] M. Donbrow, S. Benita and A. Hoffman, *Appl. Biochem. Biotechnol.*, **10**, 245 (1984).
[4] D. Babay, A. Hoffman and S. Benita, *Biomaterials*, **9**, 255 (1988).
[5] A. M. Fouili, A,. A. Sayed and A. A. Bodawi, *Int. J. Pharm.*, **14**, 95 (1983).
[6] E. M. Ramadan, A. El-Helw and Y. El-Said, *J. Microencapsul.*, **5**, 125 (1988).
[7] M. Kaweata, S. Nakamura, S. Goto and T. Aoyama, *Chem. Pharm. Bull.*, **34**, 2618 (1986).
[8] Y. Pongpaibul, J. C. Price and C. W. Whitworth, *Drug Dev. Ind. Pharm.*, **10**, 1597 (1984).
[9] A. Sawaya, J. P. Benoit and S. Benita, *J. Pharm. Sci.*, **76**, 475 (1987).
[10] S. Benita, J. P. Benoit, F. Puisieux and C. Thies, *J. Pharm. Sci.*, **73**, 1721 (1984).

10

Controlled delivery of theophylline from methacrylic ester copolymers and computer-supported pharmacokinetic assessment

Sarat C. Chattaraj, Sudip K. Das, Saroj K. Ghosal and **Bijan K. Gupta**
Division of Pharmaceutics, Department of Pharmacy, Jadavpur University, Calcutta 700032, India

SUMMARY

Theophylline is an effective bronchodilator with moderate aqueous solubility and exhibits a potential bioequivalence problem owing to the non-reproducible rate of dissolution of the drug in gastrointestinal (GI) fluid. The benefit of prolonged release formulations is not only to limit fluctuations of the serum theophylline level during the dosing interval but also to reduce the frequency of administration. Different grades of methacrylic ester copolymers (Eudragit RS 100, RSPM, S100 and L100) were used to fabricate the microcapsules and micromatrices of theophylline. Coacervation and spray congealing techniques were followed to develop the dosage form. A new type of protective colloid, polyisobutadiene, was used to enhance the effective coacervation and deposition of the coating material on to the surface. We have investigated a series from lower to higher molecular weight polyisobutadiene. Physicochemical characterization of the dosage forms was conducted for a reproducible *in vitro* drug release profile under simulated GI conditions by continuously changing the pH of the medium from 1.2 to 7.4. The *in vitro* release studies revealed a significant control of drug release compared with conventional tablets. Scanning electron micrographic studies revealed different topographical changes with different grades of coating material and protective colloid.

INTRODUCTION

Theophylline is widely used as a bronchodilator for the treatment of asthma or obstructive pulmonary disease [1]. Significant relief of bronchospasm is usually achieved with 7–20 mg/l of theophylline in serum and toxic manifestations occur above 20–30 mg/l. The available literature also reveals circadian variation of theophylline pharmacokinetics [2]. Prolonged release dosage forms of theophylline have been developed to avoid the problems associated with a narrow range of effective blood concentration [3] and a short elimination half-life in man [4], especially in children [5]. The present study was undertaken to investigate the effect of physicochemical properties of wall-forming materials on the drug release kinetics and bioavailability of microcapsules and micromatrices. The effect of a coacervation-inducing agent on the drug release profile was also studied.

EXPERIMENTAL

Materials

Eudragit RS 100, RSPM, S 100 and L 100 were received by courtesy of Röhm Pharma GmbH, Darmstadt, FRG. Theophylline (Indian Pharmacopoeia), polyisobutadiene, acetone, trichloroethylene, cyclohexane and methylene chloride were procured commercially.

Preparation of Microcapsules

Anhydrous theophylline (100 mesh) was incorporated into a homogenous 5% w/w solution of the corresponding Eudragit in its solvent (Table 1) containing 2–7% w/w of polyisobutadiene. The phase separation and subsequent deposition of the polymer was effected by desolvating the polymer (Table 1) under stirred conditions. Hardening of the microcapsules was effected by dropwise addition of the chilled non-solvent. After the formation of embryonic microcapsules, they were separated, washed with chilled non-solvent and air dried at ambient temperature.

Three batches were made and the content of drug was determined.

Table 1 — Polymer systems investigated

Polymer	Non-solvent	Solvent
Eudragit RS 100	Trichloroethylene	Cyclohexane
Eudragit RSPM	Trichloroethylene	Cyclohexane
Eudragit S 100	Acetone	Methylene Chloride
Eudragit L 100	Acetone	Methylene Chloride

Preparation of Micromatrices

Anhydrous theophylline was dispersed into a 12% w/v homogenous sol of Eudragit in a suitable solvent. This mixture was poured at 10°C, in a thin stream, into 400 ml of light mineral oil (absolute viscosity, 95–105 cP at 10°C), while stirring the system at

400±10 rev/min. After 20 min, suitable non-solvent (Table 1) was added dropwise to effect hardening of the particles.

Micromatrices were recovered from the system by filtration and successive washing with suitable non-solvent (Table 1) and dried in air.

In vitro dissolution

Drug release profiles of micromatrices and microcapsules were evaluated using a modified USP XXI dissolution apparatus under changing pH conditions. A pH profile [6] from 1.2 to 7.5 was achieved using hydrochloric acid, anhydrous sodium carbonate and bicarbonate in distilled water. Micromatrices and microcapsules were taken in the dissolution basket covered with 100 mesh muslin cloth. Initially, 500 ml of dissolution fluid was used and 5 ml aliquots were removed at specified time intervals to evaluate the percentage of drug released. The dissolved drug was assayed at 271 nm using a UV–visible 200-20 Hitachi spectrophotometer (Table 2).

Table 2 — *In vitro* drug release profile of microcapsules and micromatrices

Dosage form	Polymer material	Drug content (%)	Wall thickness µm)	T (50% min)
Microcapsules	Eudragit RS 100	82.50	14.38	110
(particle size $\bar{x}$=540 µm)	Eudragit RSPM	83.20	12.40	95
	Eudragit S 100	92.70	10.75	68
	Eudragit L 100	90.64	7.26	50
Micromatrices	Eudragit RS 100	98.20		170
(particle size $\bar{x}$=770 µm	Eudragit RSPM	95.80		154
	Eudragit S 100	89.32		96
	Eudragit L 100	87.62		70

Core:coat=1:2.

Scanning electron microscopy

As the developed dosage forms are transparent to the electron beam, the samples were coated with (carbon–gold)–gold layer under vacuum. An ISA-60A scanning electron microscope and a polar vapour coater unit were for gold coating.

In vivo evaluation

Six healthy volunteers, three males and three females, aged 20–25 years, and weighing 50–60 kg, participated in the study. Female volunteers were non-pregnant. All subjects were non-smokers. After informed consent was obtained, all subjects refrained from tea, coffee, carbonated beverage and chocolate for six days before and during the study.

The subjects fasted overnight and the developed dosage forms equivalent to 250 mg theophylline were administered at 7 a.m. with 100 ml water. The subjects were not permitted to take food until 2.5 h after dosing. Then a standardized breakfast, without tea or coffee, was given. A light meal was served at 11.30 a.m. and dinner was served at 8.30 p.m. The subjects refrained from taking any other drugs during this study. A cross-over schedule was adopted and a minimum interval of one week was allowed between each dosing. All subjects received a single oral dose of the different oral dosage forms in each schedule.

Blood samples were taken at 0.25, 0.5, 1.5, 2.5, 4.5, 6.5, 8.5, 10.5 and 12.5 h and the concentration of theophylline in serum was assayed by a spectrophotometric method [7]. The samples were analysed in duplicate. Bioavailability was calculated from the area under the concentration curve following the trapezoidal rule.

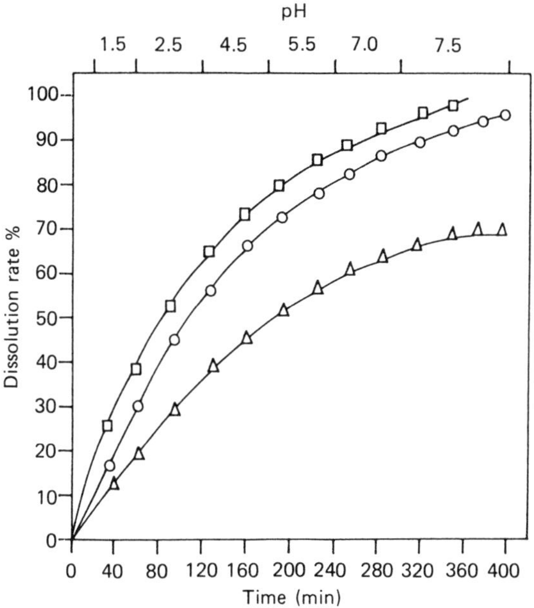

Fig. 1 — Effect of polyisobutadiene concentration on *in vitro* release of theophylline microcapsules (theophylline:RS 100 ratio, 1:2; particle size ($\bar{x}$), 540 μm): □, 2.5% (w/w); ○, 3.0% (w/w); △, 4.0% (w/w).

RESULTS AND DISCUSSION

Scanning electron micrography of the micromatrices revealed that the products were homogeneous with corrugated surfaces and pores. Higher magnification revealed surface shrinkage. After dissolution the micromatrices did not change in shape, which suggests that the drug diffused out through the minor pores and channels.

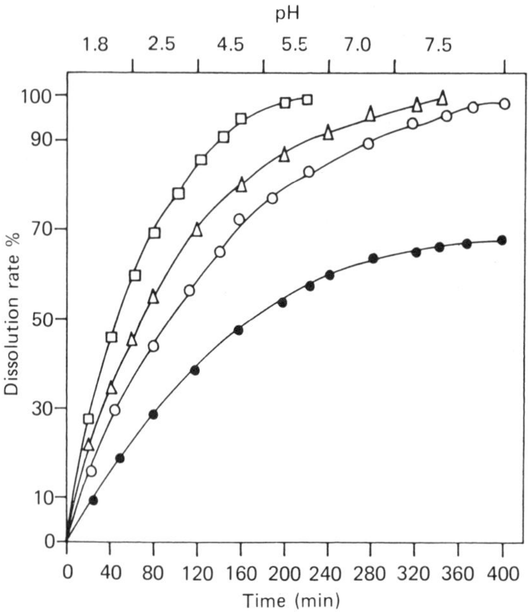

Fig. 2 — Effect of polyisobutadiene concentration on *in vitro* release of theophylline microcapsules (theophylline:RSPM ratio, 1:2; particle size ($\bar{x}$), 540 μm): □, 2.0% (w/w); △, 2.5% (w/w); ○, 3.0% (w/w); ●, 4.0% (w/w).

After being solubilized by the dissolution media. Electron micrographs of the microcapsules showed that there were a few pores on the surface of the microcapsules. Shapes were irregular owing to the amorphous nature of the drug particles used.

Lowering the viscosity of the coating medium resulted in an increased degree of aggregation of the micromatrices. Increasing the viscosity produced a higher percentage of large unacceptable micromatrices. The stirring speed was found to be the most important factor contributing to the size distribution of the micromatrices. The percentage of small particles increased at higher stirrer speed.

In vitro dissolution at increasing pH allows a comparison to be made between the different microcapsules prepared with various core:wall ratios. The drug dissolution from the microcapsules depends on the core:coat ratio and the rate of drug release decreases with a decrease in core:coat ratio.

From preliminary results, the presence of polyisobutadiene at a minimum concentration was essential for the production of free-flowing, discrete microcapsules. A concentration of polyisobutadiene of more than 2.5% was found to be suitable to give good, reproducible, microcapsules (Figs 1–3). The coacervated polymer droplet formed a smooth continuous coat around each particle, markedly different from the surface characteristics of pure drug. The mechanism of coacervated droplet stabilization could be that the polymer adsorption layers around the particles are quite dense and hence the particles undergo pseudoelastic collision, an approach rather than a mixing of their adsorption layers.

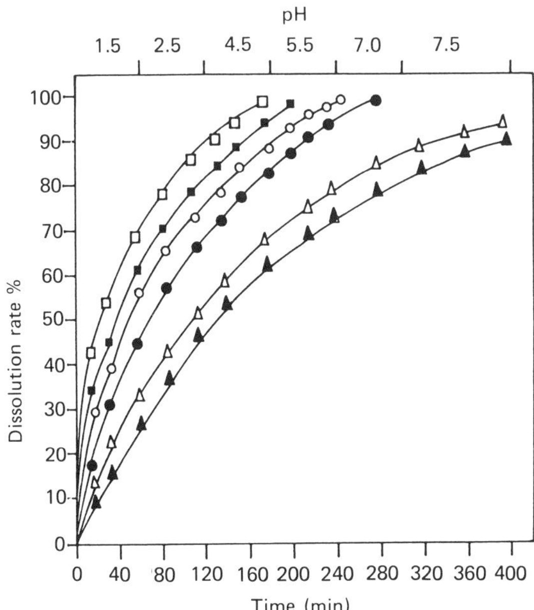

Fig. 3 — Effect of polyisobutadiene concentration on *in vitro* release of theophylline microcapsules (particle size ($\bar{x}$), 540 μm). Theophylline:S 100 ratio of 1:2: ▲, 4.0% (w/w); ●, 3.0% (w/w); ■, 2.5% (w/w). Theophylline: L 100 ratio of 1:2; △, 4.0% (w/w); ○, 3.0% (w/w); □, 2.5% (w/w).

The drug release profile was plotted against time (Figs. 4 and 5) and it was observed that the release kinetics followed both first-order and Higuchi equations up to 75–80% of the cumulative drug release. The micromatrices followed the Higuchi equation (NONLIN package).

The plasma concentration of theophylline following oral administration of Eudragit RS 100 microcapsules reached a peak at 7.1 h and decreased by a monoexponential process. This dosage form exhibited maximum prolongation. The plasma bioavailability parameters are listed in Table 3. There were significant differences in the AUC, C_{max} and T_{max} among the dosage forms. The drug release profiles of the polymers, as revealed from *in vitro* dissolution, showed correlation with the *in vivo* bioavailability parameter. Micromatrices were found to be the better dosage form for the prolongation of drug release.

Because of the pH-independent dissolution profile of Eudragit RS 100 and RSPM, the dosage forms prepared with these polymers offer better controlled release kinetics than those with S 100 and L 100, as the solubilities of the latter are pH dependent.

In conclusion, the developed controlled release dosage forms of theophylline are capable of maintaining effective therapeutic blood levels of the drug. Administration 12 hourly of these dosage forms to a healthy volunteer, gave a relatively high bioavailability, a relatively low difference between the maximum and minimum

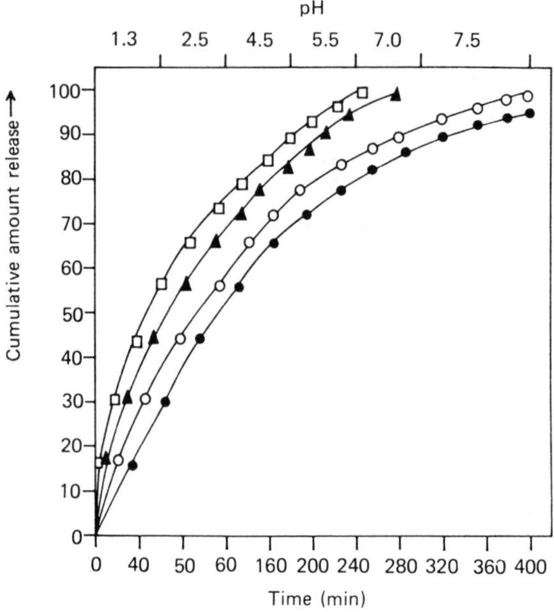

Fig. 4 — *In vitro* release profile of microcapsules (particle size ($\bar{x}$), 540 μm; core:polymer ratio, 1:2): ●, RS 100; ○, RSPM; ▲, S 100; □, L 100.

serum concentrations and a relatively small serum concentration is expected to occur provided that the dosage forms are taken in the non-fasting state.

REFERENCES

[1] L. Hendeles and M. Weinberger, *Pharmacotherapy,* **3**, 2 (1983).

[2] C. H. Feldman, V. E. Hutchinson, T. H. Sher, B. R. Feldman and W. J. Davis, *Ther. Drug Monit.,* **4**, 69 (1982).

[3] P. A. Mitenko and R. I. Ogilvie, *N. Engl., J. Med.,* **289**, 600 (1973).

[4] D. E. Zaske, K. W. Mitler, E. M. Strem, S. Austrian and P. B. Johnson, *J. Am. Med. Assoc.,* **237**, 1453 (1979).

[5] M. Weinberger, L. Hendles, L. Wong and L. Vaughan, *J. Pediatr.,* **99**, 145 (1981).

[6] S. K. Das and B. K. Gupta, *Drug Dev. Ind. Pharm.,* **14**, 537 (1988).

[7] J. Vasiliades and T. Turner, *Clin. Chim. Acta,* **69**, 491 (1976).

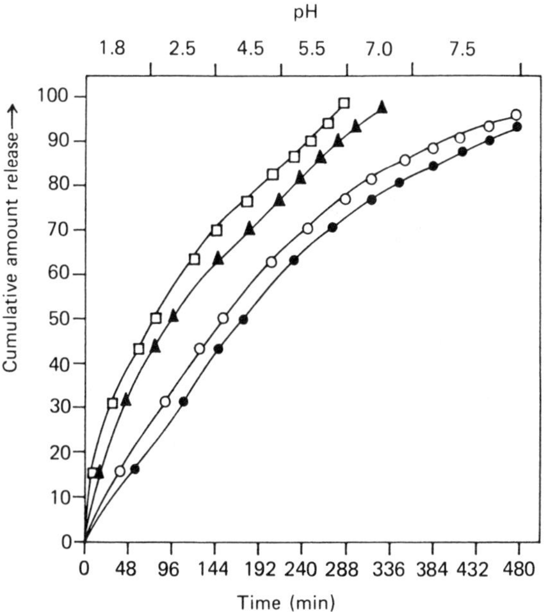

Fig. 5 — *In vitro* release profile of micromatrices (particle size ($\bar{x}$), 770 μm; core:polymer ratio, 1:2): ●, RS 100; ○, RSPM; ▲, S 100; □, L 100.

Table 3 — Pharmacokinetic parameters

Dosage form	Polymer	$AUC_{0-\infty}$ (mg/l)	C_{max}	T_{max}
Microcapsule	Eudragit RS 100	80.9	4.5	5.5
	Eudragit RSPM100	74.6	5.8	5.7
	Eudragit S 100	65.4	6.4	4.2
	Eudragit L 100	62.8	8.0	3.0
	Eudragit RS 100	84.7	3.7	7.1
	Eudragit RSPM	79.6	5.2	6.4
	Eudragit S 100	71.4	5.8	4.9
	Eudragit L 100	68.9	6.9	3.8

Each point represents the average of six results.

11

The effect of food on gastrointestinal transit and drug absorption of a multiparticular sustained release verapamil formulation

Martti Marvola, Anneli Kannikoski, Heikko Aito and **Sirkka Nykänen**
School of Pharmacy, University of Helsinki, SF-00170 Helsinki, Finland, Research Centre, Orion Pharmaceutica. SF-02101 Espoo, Finland, and Hospital of the Helsinki Deaconess Institute, SF-00530 Helsinki, Finland

INTRODUCTION

Clearly too little attention has been paid to the effect of food on drug absorption from sustained release formulations. It is still very common for adsorption studies in the drug development stage to be carried out in fasted subjects, even though, in clinical practice, fed conditions are far more usual

It is well documented that food has a clear effect on the gastrointestinal transit of single-unit controlled release products [1,2]. Even small amounts cause substantial prolongation of the gastric residence time. In contrast, the commonest claim concerning multiple-unit formulations (pellets, granules, etc.) is that food does not affect their gastric emptying rate if the diameter of the subunits is less than 2 mm [2,3].

In our previous study the gastrointestinal transit and concomitant verapamil absorption from a single-unit film-coated sustained release tablet was studied in healthy volunteers [4]. The position of the tablet in the alimentary canal at each blood sampling was detected radiographically. The results showed that food affected not only the gastrointestinal transit of the tablet but also the absorption rate of verapamil. With food, drug absorption was more rapid than under fasting conditions (t_{max} values of 8 h and 12 h respectively) since the tablet was retained for longer in the upper parts of the gastrointestinal tract, which favour drug absorption.

The aim of the present study was to repeat the experiments of the previous study using a multiple-unit verapamil formulation instead of the single-unit tablet. The *in vitro* dissolution patterns of both formulations are approximately equal, thus allowing their biopharmaceutical properties to be compared.

MATERIALS AND METHODS

Drug product

The product used was a hard gelatin capsule, size 0 (Posilok, Elanco), containing coated verapamil hydrochloride pellets (100 mg of verapamil hydrochloride) and coated barium sulphate pellets.

The verapamil pellets contained equal parts of verapamil hydrochloride (Fermion) and lactose (Ph. Eur.) plus 4% of gelatin as a binder. They were coated using a fluidized bed technique (Aeromatic Strea 1, Aeromatic AG). The coat consisted of ethyl cellulose (Ethocel N-50), Hercules) and 20% of dibutyl sebacate (E. Merck) as a plasticizer. The calculated amount of coating in the pellets was 10%. The density of the verapamil pellets was 1.13. The *in vitro* dissolution pattern was determined according to the USP paddle method; 50% of the drug was dissolved at 4.2 h.

Barium sulphate pellets were prepared using the same procedure. The ratio of barium sulphate (Barisulf-HD, Leiras) to lactose was 3:5 and the density of the barium sulphate pellets 1.35. The 0.7–1.7 mm (mean, 1.2 mm) fraction was used from both coated pellets. The volumetric ratio of verapamil pellets to barium sulphate pellets in the final formulation was 1:2.

Absorption test

Six healthy male volunteers aged 21–30 years and weighing 65–85 kg were informed about the possible risks and side effects of the study and their written consent was obtained. Routine clinical tests showed all subjects to have values within the normal ranges. The Ethical Committee of the Helsinki Deaconess Institute Hospital approved the experimental protocol.

The cross-over study was carried out in two parts. In the first part the subjects were fasted overnight and at 8 a.m. took one capsule with 100 ml of tap water. Food was subsequently withheld for 3 h, after which a standard lunch was served. Blood was sampled (10 ml) just before and 2, 4, 8, 12, 24 and 32 h after dosage. Immediately following each blood sample (except at 0 and 32 h) an X-ray photograph was taken to determine the position of the pellets in the gastrointestinal tract. The X-ray photographs were taken in the supine position and the sites of the alimentary canal numbered as in Table 1.

One week later the test was repeated under non-fasting conditions. Just before drug administration a standard heavy breakfast was served consisting of oatmeal porridge (400 g), cheese (40 g), orange juice (100 ml) and coffee or tea (200 ml). A standard lunch was served 3 h later.

Verapamil and its active metabolite norverapamil were assayed from serum (frozen at −18°C) using a gas chromatographic–mass spectrometric method [5]. The detection limit of the method was 1 ng/ml. The areas under the concentration–time curves (AUC 0–32 h) were calculated by the trapezoidal method. Statistical evaluation was carried out using the paired Wilcoxon test and paired Student's *t* test.

RESULTS

A summary of the gastrointestinal transit in all six volunteers is given in Fig. 1. The position of the pellets furthest down in the gastrointestinal tract was numbered

Table 1 — Number codes for different parts of the gastrointestinal tract

Number	Anatomical part
1	Stomach
2	Duodenum
3	Jejunum
4	Ileum
5	Terminal ileum
6	Ascendent colon
7	Transverse colon
8	Descendant colon
9	Sigmoid colon
10	Rectum

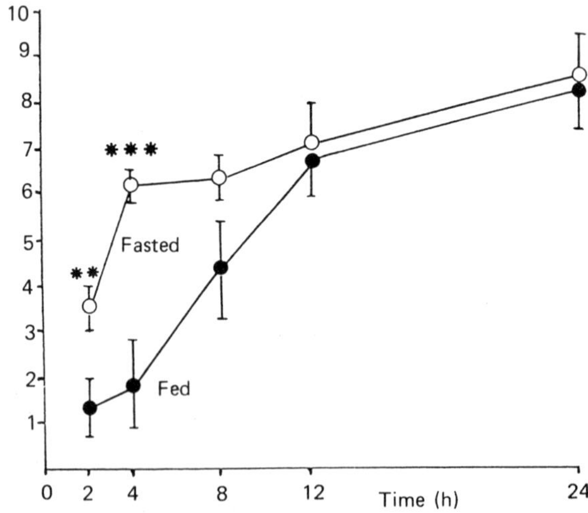

Fig. 1 — Passage of ethylcellulose-coated pellets through the gastrointestinal tract in six healthy volunteers. The position of the foremost part of the dose has been numbered according to Table 1. Each point represents the mean ±SD. **, $p<0.01$; ***, $p<0.001$.

according to Table 1. Fig. 1 shows that food taken just before drug administration clearly delayed gastric emptying of the pellets up to 8 h. The differences were statistically significant at 2 and 4 h ($p;<0.05$).

Examination of the results on the basis of where the majority of pellets were situated (Table 2) shows that food increased the gastric residence time in each volunteer by 2–10 h. The entry of most pellets into the colon was usually delayed from 4 to 12 h, but in one case (JO) for more than 18 h (Table 3).

Table 2 — Radiological evaluation of the time during which the majority of pellets were retained in the stomach

Experimental conditions	Volunteer					
	JA	MH	PJ	KM	JO	MT
Fasting	2	<2	<2	2	2	<2
Non-fasting	8	4	8	4	12	8

Table 3 — Radiological evaluation of the time during which the majority of the pellets had entered the colon

Experimental conditions	Volunteer					
	JA	MH	PJ	KM	JO	MT
Fasting	12	8	4	4	8	12
Non-fasting	24	12	12	12	>24	24

Fig. 2 shows the serum verapamil levels of each volunteer in both the fasted and the fed states, and the position of the majority of pellets at each blood sampling. Especially large differences in time–concentration curves were noted if in the fasted state the majority of pellets had already entered the intestine at 2 h but in the fed state remained in the stomach for more than 4 h (volunteers KM and TM).

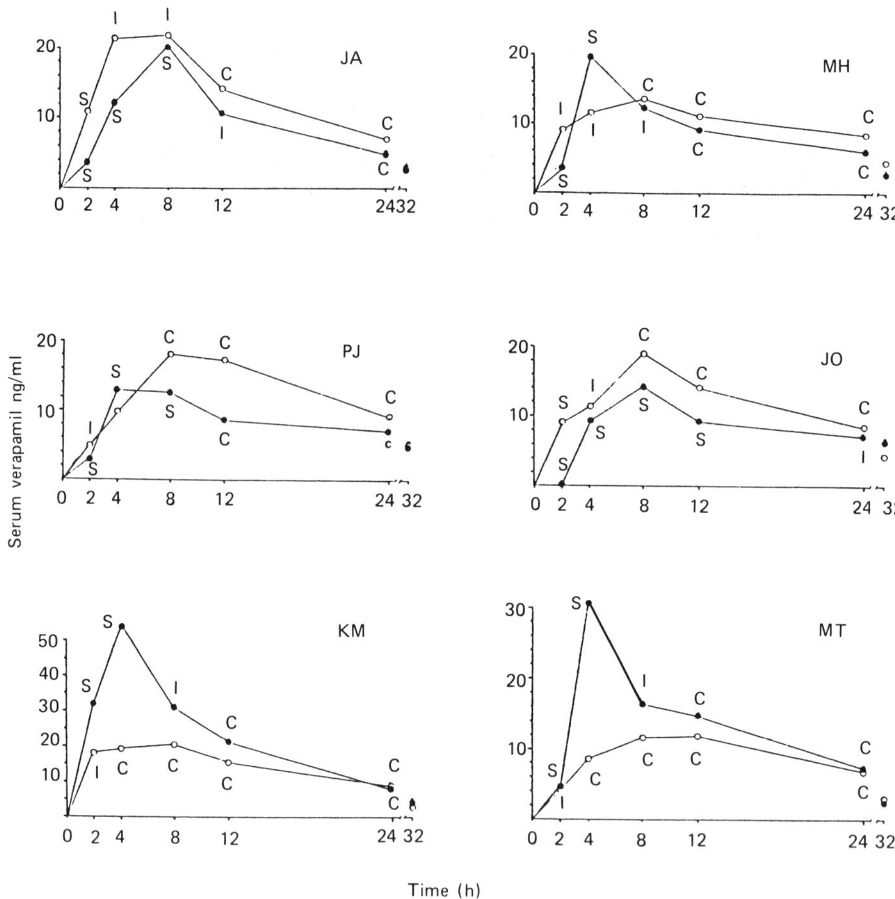

Fig. 2 — Absorption of verapamil after a single dose of a sustained release pellet formulation in six healthy volunteers. The position of the majority of pellets at each blood sampling was detected by X-rays. S, stomach; I, intestine; C, colon; ○, fasting; ●, non-fasting.

CONCLUSION

We conclude that food, and especially a heavy meal, markedly enhances the gastric residence time of pellets administered in a hard gelatin capsule. Clearly most of the pellets were only swept out of the stomach by the migrating motor complex ('housekeeper wave'). This delay in gastric emptying can cause a higher and earlier peak in blood drug concentration, leading to some side effects. Thus it is important that in the development of modified release formulations, both single unit and multiple unit, bioavailability studies should be carried out under both fasting and non-fasting conditions. Testing a light breakfast only may be misleading. According to the results of absorption studies, patients must also be informed on the proper timing of drug administration in relation to meals.

REFERENCES

[1] A. Cortot and J. Colombel. *Int. J. Pharm.*, **22**, 321–325 (1984).
[2] S. Davies, J. Hardy and J. Fara, *Gut,* **27**, 886–892 (1986).
[3] S. O'Reilly, C. Wilson and J. Hardy, *Int. J. Pharm.*, **34**, 213–216 (1987).
[4] M. Marvola, H. Aito, P. Pohto, A. Kannikoski, S. Nykänen and P. Kokkonen, *Drug Dev. Ind. Pharm.*, **13**, 1593–1609 (1987).
[5] M. Marvola, A. Kannikoski, J. Taskinen and P. Ottoila, *J. Pharm. Pharmacol.*, **37**, 766–770 (1985).

12

Biodegradable polymers: Effect of thermal treatment on the physicomechanical and dissolution properties of compacts

Marcelo O. Omelczuk
Drug Dynamics Institute, College of Pharmacy, The University of Texas at Austin, Austin, TX 78712-1074 USA
Kuei-Tu Chang
Sterling-Winthrop Research Institute, Rensselaer, NY 12144-3493 NY
and
James W. McGinity
Drug Dynamics Institute, College of Pharmacy, The University of Texas at Austin, Austin, TX 78712-1074 USA

SUMMARY

Biodegradable polymers, such as poly(lactic acid) and poly(caprolactone), were investigated as binders in the formulation of matrix tablets for controlled release. Polymers of different stereo configuration and molecular weights were incorporated into tablet formulations containing the model drug theophylline in combination with excipients such as microcrystalline cellulose. It was shown that thermal treatment of these tablets above the glass transition temperature of the polymer accelerated, retarded or had an insignificant effect on the dissolution release rate of theophylline from the compact, as compared with the non-thermally treated tablets.

INTRODUCTION

Polymers, such as poly(lactic acid) and poly(caprolactone), have been classified as being biocompatible or biodegradable. *In vivo*, these polymers eventually undergo hydrolytic scission, producing by products which can be metabolically handled by the body. For example, poly(lactic acid) is susceptible to hydrolytic de-esterification to lactic acid, a normal metabolite in the glycolytic in carbohydrate metabolism [1,2].

Other important properties include their non-toxicity, sterilizability and stability. These polymers can also be cast into films and are completely miscible with many other polymers and plasticizers. Perhaps the most important characteristic is that they can be synthetically engineered to produce desirable chemical, physical and mechanical properties. To date, most of these polymers have been investigated for use in surgical repair materials [1,3]. Other promising areas of application have involved the use of these polymers in developing systems for implication, injection, and insertion [2,5–7]. The use of these polymers in these areas offers the advantage of tissue compatibility and negates the need for surgical removal. Current investigations using these polymers have begun to focus on the potential applications in controlled release transdermal systems, tablets, pellets and microspheres, as well as for controlled release coating formulations [5–9]. In the present investigation, the primary objective was to study the dissolution release properties of tablets containing poly(lactic acid) and poly(caprolactone), when utilized as binders in matrix tablets for controlled release.

EXPERIMENTAL

Preliminary studies have investigated tablet formulations using low molecular weight L-poly(lactic acid) (L-PLA) and DL-poly(lactic acid) (DL-PLA), as well as high molecular weight DL-PLA and poly(caprolactone) (PCL-300 and 700). Formulations were made containing 25% and 60% anhydrous theophylline (Sigma Chemicals, St. Louis, MO), 15% polymer and excipient (microcrystalline cellulose, Avicel PH-101, FMC Corporation, Philadelphia, PA). The model drug theophylline was mixed with the excipient for 10 min in a twin-shell blender. The polymers were incorporated into the tablet formulations as binder solutions by dissolving the polymer in methylene chloride to a concentration of 20–30%. A wet granulation process was then used to distribute the polymer solution or dispersion into the powder blend of the model drug theophylline and the excipient. The granulations were then air dried overnight at 25°C and passed through a 20 mesh screen. Tablets weighing 300 mg were compressed to a tablet hardness of 10–12 kg. Samples of these tablets were then heated at 60°C for 24 h and allowed to equilibrate to room temperature for 12 h. Some tablets containing high molecular weight DL-PLA were also heated for 24 h at 40°C, and for 1 and 12 h at 60°C. Tablets were also prepared from aqueous latex dispersions of the DL-PLA. Dissolution studies were preformed on both the thermally and the non-thermally treated tablets in water at 37°C, using the USP XXI method 2. Paddle speed was 50 rev/min. Samples of the dissolution medium were taken periodically and analysed by UV spectroscopy (Beckman DU spectrophotometer) at a wavelength of 270 nm for theophylline.

Molecular weight was determined using gel permeation chromatography (GPC, Waters Millipore). The glass transition temperatures (T_g) were analysed using differential scanning calorimetry (Perkin–Elmer DSC-2).

RESULTS AND DISCUSSION

The data in Table 1 provide a comparison of molecular weights, molecular weight distributions and glass transition temperatures of the different polymers used in the

Table 1 — Polymer characteristics

	M_n	M_w	M_w/M_n	T_g(°C)
L-Poly(lactic acid) (L-PLA (LMW))	1103	3080	2.80	24
DL-Poly(lactic acid) (DL-PLA (LMW))	1296	3035	2.34	27
DL-Poly(lactic acid) (DL-PLA (HMW))	52000	110000	2.12	57
Poly(caprolactone) (PCL-300)	18800	30400	1.62	−65
Poly(caprolactone) (PCL-700)	47000	90700	1.94	−65

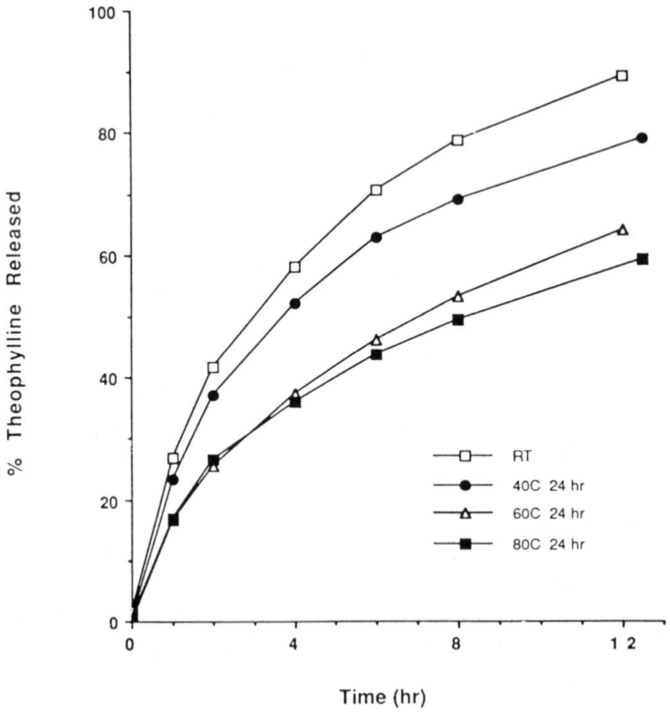

Fig. 1 — Influence of thermal treatment on the drug release from tablets containing 15% HMW DL-PLA, 25% theophylline and 60% microcrystalline cellulose.

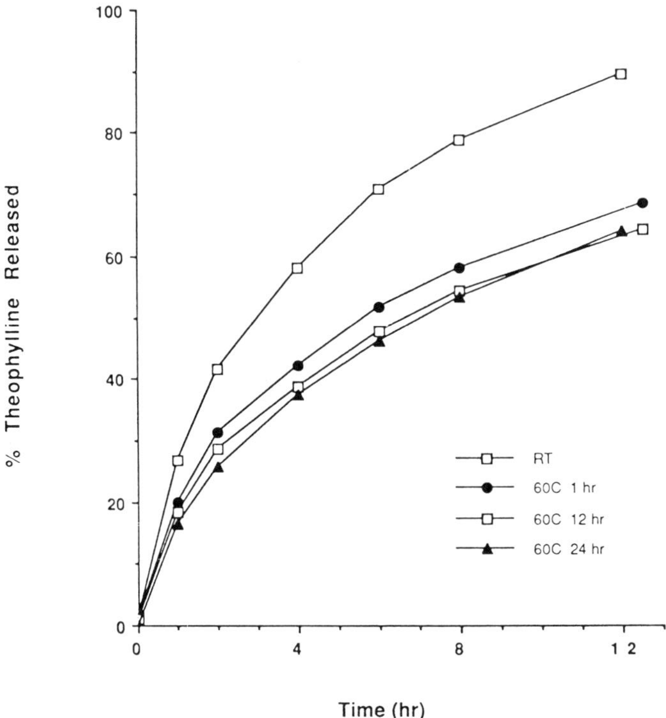

Fig. 2 — Influence of the duration of thermal treatment on the drug release from tablets containing 15% HMW, DL-PLA, 25% theophylline and 60% microcrystalline cellulose.

various tablet formulations. When tablets containing 25% drug and 15% high molecular weight DL-PLA were heated above the glass transition temperature of the polymer (57°C), a significant retardation of drug release was found when compared with the tablets heated below this temperature (Fig. 1).Furthermore, the longer the duration of thermal treatment, the greater the retardation of drug release when compared with the non-thermally treated tablets, as shown in Fig. 2. However, relative to 1 h thermal treatment, the retardation in drug release became less pronounced as the duration of thermal treatment was increased to 12 and 24 h.

Although the non-heated tablets did not disintegrate, they did partially split on their horizontal axis after a few minutes in the dissolution medium. In contrast, the thermally treated tablets remained totally intact. This splitting phenomenon of the non-thermally treated tablets increased the surface area of the tablet which could contribute to the more rapid dissolution rate of drug as compared with the thermally treated tablets. The tablet formulation also contains 60% microcrystalline cellulose as the filler. At this concentration, microcrystalline cellulose can act as a wicking agent which may promote disintegration of the tablet matrix [10]. However, the binding capacity of the high molecular weight DL-PLA in the thermally treated tablets appeared to counteract the disintegration effect of microcrystalline cellulose

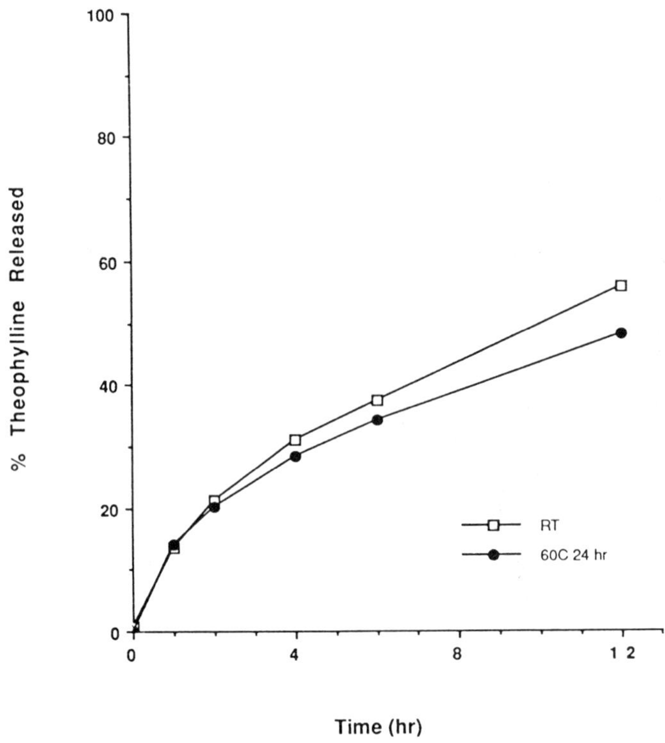

Fig. 3 — Influence of thermal treatment on the drug release from tablets containing 15% HMW DL-PLA, 60% theophylline and 25% microcrystalline cellulose.

and to hold the tablet matrix intact. Compaction studies demonstrated that the thermally treated tablets were significantly harder than the non-thermally treated tablets, which suggested better binding. Thus, it is possible that thermal treatment increases the binding capacity within the tablet resulting in a slower release rate of drug from the tablet matrix, especially above the glass transition temperature of the polymer.

Dissolution profiles from tablets containing 60% theophylline and 25% microcrystalline cellulose showed a smaller difference in the release rate of theophylline from heated and non-heated tablets (Fig. 3). Nevertheless, both of these tablets demonstrated a matrix-controlled release. These results suggest that the level of excipient in the tablet exerted a significant effect on the dissolution release properties of thermally and non-thermally treated tablets. As the microcrystalline cellulose content increased, the difference in release rates between heated and non-heated tablets became more pronounced.

Dissolution studies were also conducted on tablets containing high molecular weight PCL-300 and PCL-700 (Fig. 4). As with the high molecular weight DL-PLA formulations, there was a significant retardation in release rate of theophylline from thermally treated tablets when compared with the non-thermally treated tablets.

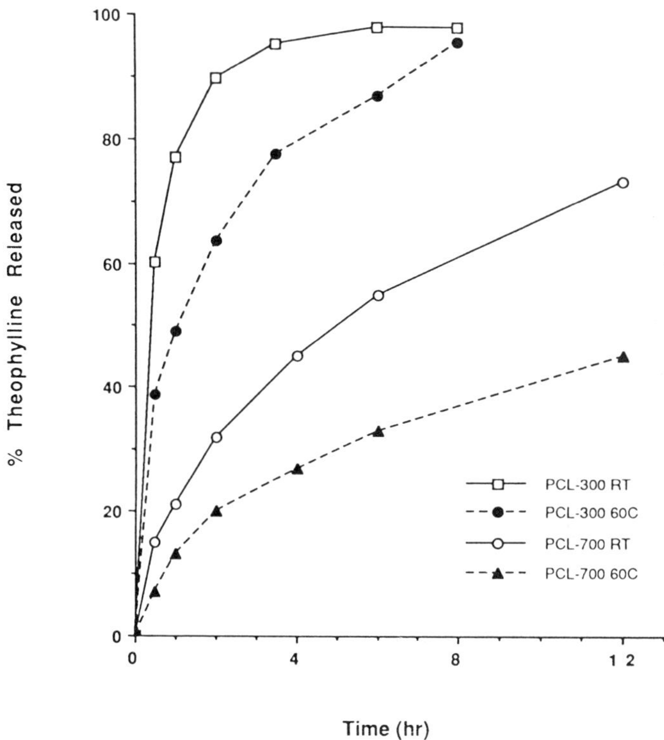

Fig. 4 — Influence of thermal treatment on the drug release from tablets containing 15% PCL-300 and 700, 25% theophylline and 60% microcrystalline cellulose.

The data in Figs 5 and 6 show dissolution profiles of theophylline from tablets containing low molecular weight DL-PLA. These profiles demonstrated that there was no significant difference in the dissolution release rate between the heated and non-heated tablets for both the 25% and the 60% theophylline formulations. In all cases, the tablets disintegrated within minutes and 100% of the theophylline was released within 1 h. These results suggested that, regardless of the thermal treatment, low molecular DL-PLA had less of a binding capacity than the high molecular weight DL-PLA. Although thermal treatment increased the hardness of the tablet, it still rapidly disintegrated in water at 37°C. Dissolution studies were conducted at 37°C, which is above the glass transition temperature of the low molecular weight DL-PLA. The T_g of this polymer is 27°C. Above the glass transition temperature, the chains of the polymer become more flexible and may loosen the binding capacity of the polymer in the tablet matrix, as evidenced by the rapid disintegration of the tablets when exposed to water at 37°C.

The dissolution profiles in Figs 7 and 8 for theophylline tablets containing a low molecular weight L-PLA, microcrystalline cellulose, and theophylline. Thermal treatment had no significant effect on the dissolution profiles from tables containing 25% theophylline (Fig. 7). As with the tablets containing low molecular weight DL-

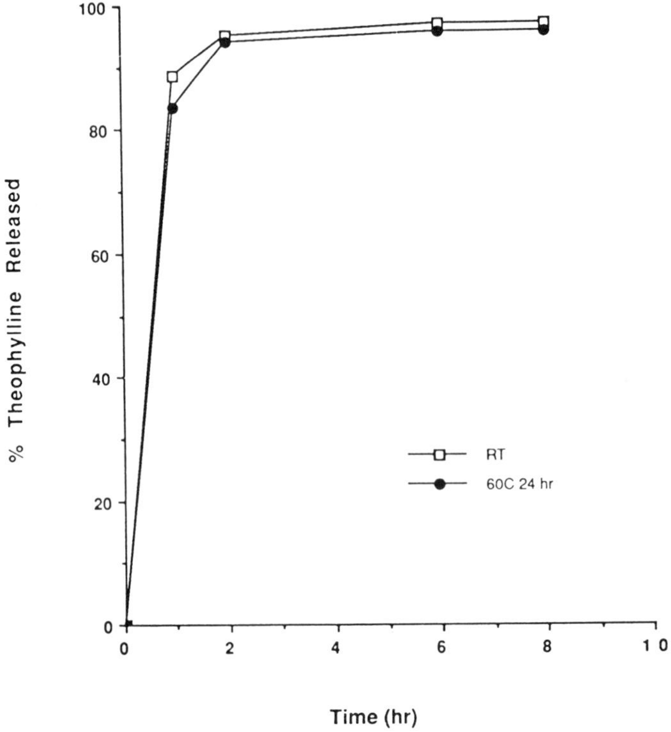

Fig. 5 — Influence of thermal treatment on the drug release from tablets containing 15% LMW DL-PLA, 25% theophylline and 60% microcrystalline cellulose.

PLA, these tablets disintegrated rapidly, releasing 100% theophylline within 1 h. However, the dissolution rate of theophylline from tablets containing 60% drug was accelerated from the thermally treated tablets when compared with the non-thermally treated tablets (Fig. 8). Although these tablets disintegrated within hours, the thermally treated tablets disintegrated faster then the non-thermally treated tablets. Low molecular weight L-PLA degrades rapidly at high temperatures, which may explain the rapid release of drug from the heat-treated tablets. This degradation of polymer, causing a decrease in moleular weight, may produce changes in the physicomechanical properties of the polymer, such as altering the degree of crystallinity and lowering the glass transition temperature. This is turn may promote faster disintegration of the tablet matrix when exposed to temperatures above the polymer glass transition temperature.

CONCLUSIONS

Thermally treated tablets containing high molecular weight DL-PLA and PCL-300 demonstrated a retardation in the dissolution release rate of theophylline from tablet compacts containing 60% microcrystalline cellulose, while thermally treated tablets

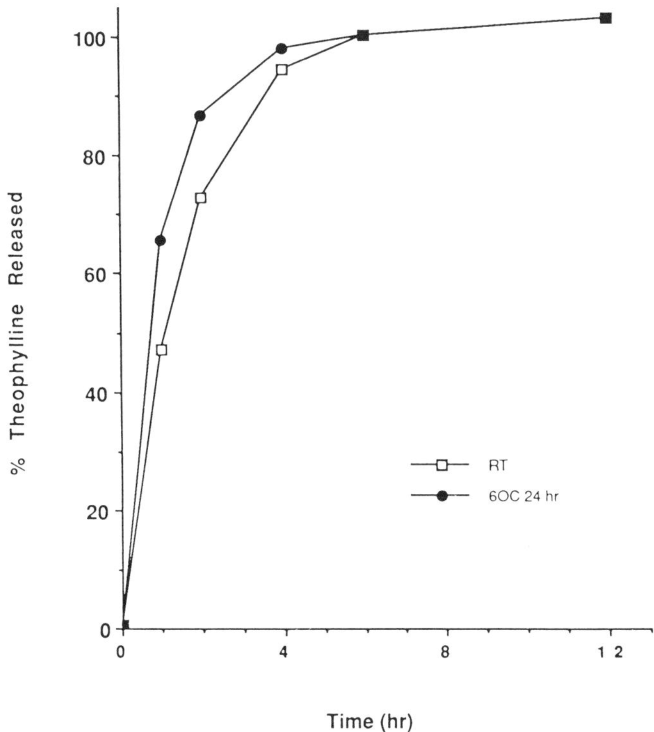

Fig. 6 — Influence of thermal treatment on the drug release from tablets containing 15% LMW DL-PLA, 60% theophylline and 25% microcrystalline cellulose.

containing low molecular DL-PLA showed no significant change in the drug dissolution rate when compared with non-thermally treated tablets. In contrast, tablets containing low molecular weight L-PLA showed an acceleration in the dissolution rate after thermal treatment. These results suggest that the physicochemical properties of the polymers, in combination with thermal treatment, have a significant effect on the dissolution rate when incorporated into these tablet formulations. Polymers with high molecular weight may act as better binders and promote the retardation of the dissolution rate of tablets after thermal treatment. However, our preliminary results also suggest that the ratio of drug to excipient and the properties of the excipient may also exert a significant influence on the retardation mechanism of thermally treated compacts.

REFERENCES

[1] R. K. Kulkarni, E. G. Moore, A. F. Hegyeli and F. Leonard, *J. Biomed. Mater. Res.*, **5**, 169 (1971).

[2] M. Anderson and F. Gibbons, *Biomater., Med. Dev., Ary, Org.*, **2**(3), 235 (1974).

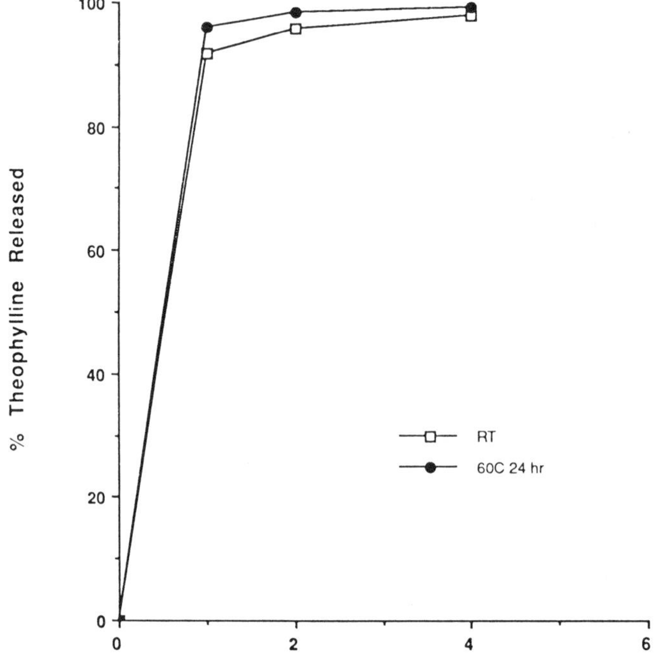

Fig. 7 — Influence of thermal treatment on the drug release from tablets containing 15% LMW L-PLA, 25% theophylline and 60% microcrystalline cellulose.

[3] S. Yolles and M. F. Sartori, in A. Kydonieus (ed.), *Controlled Release Technology: Erodible Matrices*, CRC Press, Boca Raton, 1980, p. 1.

[4] B. Farhadieh, Ŝ. Borodkin and J. D. Buddenhagen, *J. Pharm. Sci.*, **60**, 209 (1971).

[5] C. G. Pitt, M. M. Gratzl, A. R. Jeffcoat and R. Zweidinger, *J. Pharm. Sci.*, **68**, 1534 (1979).

[6] J. Heller and R. W. Baker, *Theory and Practice of Controlled Drug Delivery from Biodegradable Polymers*, Academic Press, New York, 1980.

[7] A. Schindler, J. F. Kimble and G. Pitt, *Contemporary Topics in Polymer Science*, Vol. 2, Plenum, New York, 1977, p. 271.

[8] R. Bodmier and J. W. McGinity, *Pharm. Res.*, **4**, 465 (1987).

[9] R. Chang, J. Price and C. Whitworth, *Drug Dev. Ind. Pharm.* **12**(14), 2355 (1986).

[10] *Handbook of Pharmaceutical Excipients*, Vol. 1, American Pharmacetical Association, Washington, DC, 1986, p. 53.

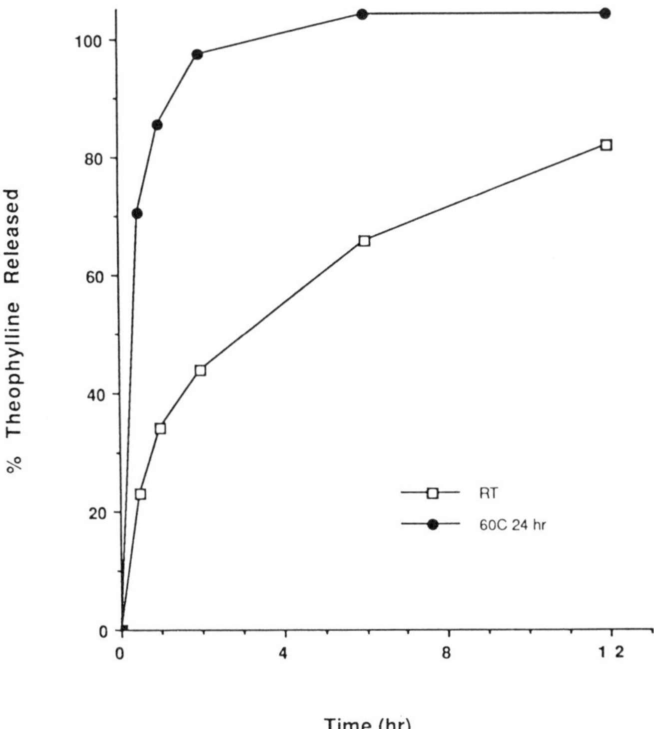

Fig. 8 — Influence of thermal treatment on the drug release from tablets containing 15% LMW L-PLA, 60% theophylline and 25% microcrystalline cellulose.

13

A comparison of dissolution properties from matrix tablets prepared from microcapsules and mixtures containing phenobarbitone and poly(DL-lactic acid)

Biljana Oraceska, Reza Ul Jalil and **J. R. Nixon**
Chelsea Department of Pharmacy, King's College London, Manresa Road, London SW3 6LX, UK

SUMMARY

Microcapsules for use in the preparation of sustained release formulations have been under investigation for a number of years without any great success. There is an initially rapid release, due to the porosity of the wall coupled with the effect of wall saturation, which builds up during long storage. Compression has provided formulations with better sustained release characteristics.

The materials traditionally used for the walls have been non-biodegradable and this meant that only the oral route has been available.

The present study investigates a biodegradable polymer, poly(DL-lactic acid) (DL-PLA), as the microcapsule wall. Tablets of microcapsules prepared with this method should be capable of use as subcutaneous implants. Three different compression forces, 2, 5 and 10 kN, were used, with core:wall ratios of 1:1 and 2:1. For comparison, the same proportions of drug and coating polymer were compressed without prior microencapsulation.

The release of the drug phenobarbitone (PB) from tablets prepared using simple mixtures of DL-PLA and PB, as well as from the corresponding tablets from microencapsulated PB, is reported. These results are compared with release from the original microcapsules.

INTRODUCTION

Oral administration is a relatively safe route for sustained action drug delivery. Oral delivery allows the use of either tablets or capsules [1]. A wide range of techniques is available for their preparation.

The drug may be incorporated in a slowly eroding matrix of waxy materials, embedded in a plastic matrix, complexed with anion exchange resins or incorporated in a water-insoluble hydrophilic matrix. Drug release from these systems occurs by several mechanisms; diffusion, dissolution, ionic exchange or osmotic pressure [1,2], depending on the type of polymeric excipient present and the formulation used.

In most cases the polymeric excipient is the principal component of the sustained release formulations which retards drug release from the dosage form. Many hydrophilic, hydrophobic or pH-sensitive polymers have been used in oral dosage forms [3]. Poly(lactic acid) (PLA) was first suggested by Kulkarni *et al.* [4] as a suitable biodegradable polymer for surgical sutures and implant material, and Yolles *et al.* [5] made use of it as an erodible implant for the controlled release of naltrexone, a narcotic antagonist. Beck *et al.* [6,7] reported the preparation of long-acting injectable microcapsules containing a contraceptive steroid using this polymer. During the past 15 years many workers have utilized this polymer. During the past 15 years many workers have utilized this polymer to fabricate a wide range of drugs in the form of implants, microcapsules, microspheres, nanoparticles and pseudolattices [8–13].

Poly(lactide) can be synthesized from two optically isomeric forms of lactic acid: L-lactic acid [14]. The polymers prepared from these isomers, L-PLA and DL-PLA, vary considerably with respect to their physical properties (crystallinity, glass transition temperatures, water uptake, etc.) which could be crucial in a diffusion-controlled drug delivery system. Drug diffusion occurs almost exclusively through the amorphous region of the polymer, so the crystalline polymer can be regarded as providing a heterogeneous medium for diffusion [15]. As L-PLA is highly crystalline, whereas DL-PLA is almost exclusively amorphous [16], diffusion through the latter should be more rapid and also more amenable to modification. Although much work has been reported on the polymers, the use of PLA in sustained release tablet formulations is not well documented. However, Coffin *et al.* [17] reported the preparation of pseudolattices from poly (DL-lactide) which they subsequently used to prepare sustained release theophylline tablets.

In the present study we report the release of phenobarbitone (PB) from tablets derived from simple mixtures of DL-PLA and PB as well as from microencapsulated PB, and the effect of the compressive force. These results are compared with release from the original microcapsules.

EXPERIMENTAL

Materials

Poly(DL-lactic acid) (Boehringer) and phenobarbitone (Sigma) were used. All other materials were of standard reagent grade purity.

Preparation of microcapsules

Poly(DL-lactic acid) and phenobarbitone were dissolved in acetonitrile at 55°C and added to a liquid paraffin–Span 40 (50:1) mixture at the same temperature. The mixture was stirred at 2000 rev min^{-1} for 30 min and then cooled to 20°C while still stirring. The resultant microcapsules were separated by filtration, washed four times with petroleum ether (boiling point, 40–60°C), dried in a stream of nitrogen and stored in a desiccator.

Preparation of mixtures

Non-microencapsulated mixtures of poly (DL-lactic acid) and phenobarbitone (ratios 1:1 and 1:2) were prepared by mixing the powders for 10 min.

Preparation of tablets

Tablets were prepared from both the microcapsules and mixtures using a Dartec Ltd universal testing machine. The quantity of drug contained was a nominal 200 mg and the punch diameter was 10 mm. Compression was at a constant rate of 1 kN s^{-1} with tablets prepared at 2, 5 and 10 kN. The tensile strength of the tablets was calculated using the formula $T_s=2P/Dt\pi$. The characteristics of the tablets prepared are shown in Table 1.

Table 1 — Characteristics of tablets prepared from microcapsules and mixtures of polymer and drug

System	Drug: polymer ratio	Mean tablet mass (mg)	Mean drug content (mg)	Compressive force (kN)	Tensile strength
Microcapsules	1:1	387.2	160.7	2	3.89
		374.2	155.3	5	4.10
		365.2	151.6	10	4.25
	2:1	306.0	182.7	2	2.88
		289.0	172.5	5	3.20
		299.6	178.9	10	3.57
Mixtures	1:1	398.0	199.0	2	0.77
		397.0	198.5	5	1.29
		392.3	196.2	10	1.61
	2:1	304.0	202.6	2	0.37
		261.0	174.6	5	0.54
		287.0	191.3	10	1.11

Particle size measurements

A Coulter counter (model TA II) attached to an Apple computer (IIe) was used for all particle size measurements.

Scanning electron microscopy

A scanning electron microscope (Philips 501B) was used to examine both microcapsules and mixtures, as well as the surface characteristics of the tablets prepared from them.

Dissolution studies

The computerized automatic dissolution apparatus utilized a Philips P118620 UV spectrophotometer connected to an Opus PC III computer. Aqueous buffer (1 l; pH 2, 7 or 9) was used at a temperature of 37±0.5°C and a stirring rate of 100 rev min^{-1}. Read-out was every 5 min for 2 h at pH 2, every 30 min for 6 h at pH 7 and every 60 min for 12 h at pH 9.

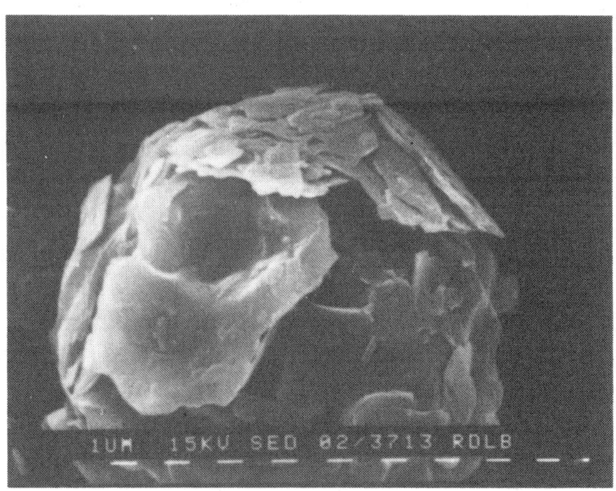

Fig. 1 — Scanning electron micrograph of an individual microcapsule showing plates of DL-PLA on the surface (core:coat ratio, 1:1).

RESULTS AND DISCUSSION

The appearance of the individual microcapsules is shown in Fig. 1. Most individual microcapsules are approximately spherical and show a surface made up of deposited plates of poly(DL-lactic acid) in which the drug is embedded. Many of the larger microcapsules are cemented together by further plates of poly(DL-lactic acid). The effect of compression on these microcapsules is shown in Fig. 2. At a compressive force of 2 kN (Fig. 2(a)) the electron micrograph of the tablet fracture surface shows that the microcapsules, while distorted, remain essentially intact and rounded, with a relatively open porous structure to the tablet as a whole. At 10 kN force (Fig. 2(b)) the microcapsules at the fracture are flattened, cracked and distorted so that the fracture surface shows a far less open, porous aspect. Both of these 'microcap' tablets have a very different appearance from that produced by the simple mixture (Fig. 3), where the individual plates of poly(DL-lactic acid) are mixed with the drug crystals in an open structure from which release would be easily accomplished. The voids and wide pores between the polymer matrix which exist after dissolution are clearly visible in Fig. 4.

Release of the drug from individual microcapsules is extremely rapid, irrespective of pH or the drug:polymer wall ratio. At pH 7 and 9 it is complete within 5 min. Even at pH 2 release was complete after 2 h. The kinetics approximated to first-order release at pH 2, but dissolution was too rapid at the higher pH values to assess the kinetics.

Particle size distribution, on a population basis, presented a predominantly unimodal distribution, with a mean size of 26.53 μm for 1:1 ratio microcapsules and 50.29 μm for 2:1 ratio systems. On a population basis the number of aggregates is small, although some of those produced from the 2:1 core:wall systems were 200–300 μm.

While the individual microcapsules did not produce any significant sustained release action, compression into tablets allowed the production of a significantly extended release. The effect of using poly(DL-lactic acid)-coated microcapsules rather than simple mixtures was also investigated.

With a drug:polymer ratio of 1:1 release from the 'microcap' tablets into pH 2 buffer was slow and there was little difference between the three compressive forces over the 2 h period (Table 2). However, when the drug:polymer ratio was raised to 2:1, differences were observed between tablets compressed at 2 kN and those at 5 and 10 kN, the latter showing almost the same release characteristics. These tablets all showed more release than from the 1:1 ratio systems. Tablets prepared from drug–polymer mixtures to give matrix tablets were compared with the 'microcap' tablets and showed a far more rapid release than the corresponding tablet. After 30 min the 1:1 ratio matrix tablet had released the same amount of drug at pH 2, irrespective of the compression, but from this time divergences began to appear, with the lowest compression tablets releasing most drug and with little significant difference between those produced at the two higher forces. A similar pattern was evident with the 2:1 ratio matrix tablets. Again, the lowest compression released more rapidly.

At pH 7 the amount of drug released was significantly higher in all cases, reflecting the increased drug solubility; 2.625 g l^{-1} as against 1.89 g l^{-1} at pH 2. Even with a 1:1 ratio 'microcap' tablet, compression effects are shown. A slightly increased release existed at the higher compression, which is contrary to that found with the 2:1 ratio systems where the lowest compression allowed a significantly faster release than with the two higher compression forces. The latter trend is also shown by both ratios of matrix-type tablets at this dissolution pH, as also is the higher drug quantity released.

At pH 9 there is a further slight increase in the amount which is released, over that from the two lower pH values, at all three compression forces. However, the same release patterns hold, with more being released after lower compression force and a higher amount from the matrix as against the 'microcap' tablet. Only with the latter type, at a ration of 1:1, is this trend not followed and, as at other pH values, with this system there appears to be only an insignificant effect of compression.

The values in Table 2 represent the actual amounts (mg) released from the systems but, if the released percentage of the drug available is compared, a slightly different picture emerges, as shown in Figs 5 and 6. A Higuchi plot (percentage released vs. $t^{1/2}$) indicates matrix release kinetics at all compressions and pH values

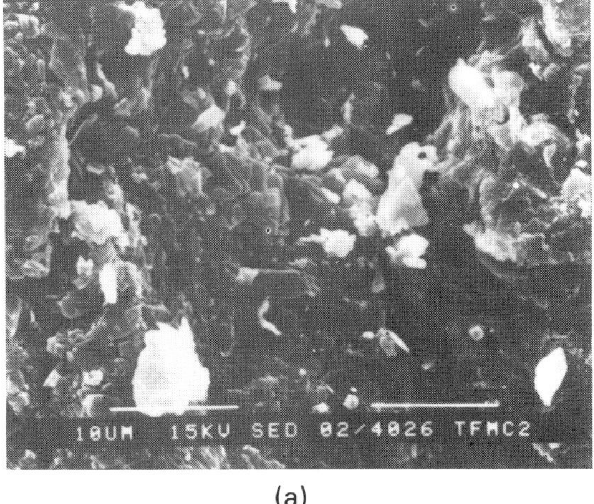

(a)

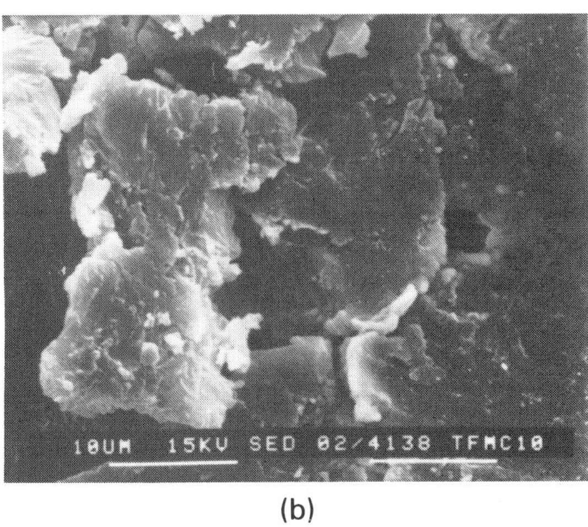

(b)

Fig. 2 — (a) Scanning electron micrograph of the tablet fracture surface from a 'microcap' tablet. Compressive force, 2 kN; core:coat ratio, 1:1. The photograph shows that microcapsules had only slightly broken down. (b) Scanning electron micrograph of the tablet fracture surface from a 'microcap' tablet. Compressive force, 10 kN; core:coat ratio, 1:1. The photograph shows compressed and broken microcapsules.

with both 'microcap' and simple matrix tablets. All systems show a short lag phase before a steady release rate is reached.

At pH 2 (Fig. 5) the 'microcap' tablets show a very much slower release than the matrix mixture systems irrespective of compression. The 2:1 core:wall microcap tablets release at more than double the rate of the 1:1 systems, but the effect of increased compression was slight and only a small fall in release rate occurred at 10 kN. A far more significant difference was noticeable with the matrices. Here the

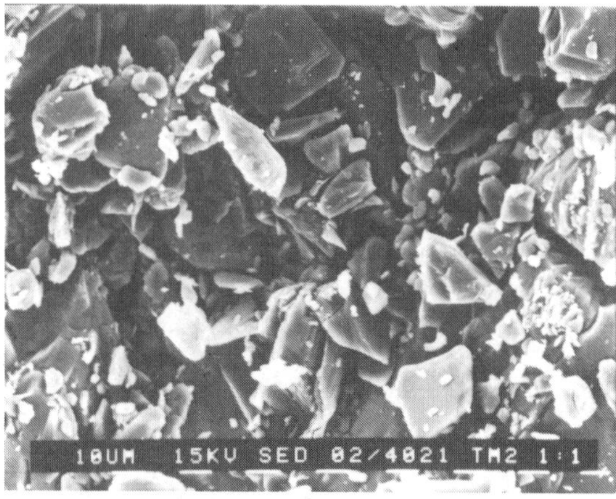

Fig. 3 — Scanning electron micrograph of the tablet fracture surface from a 'matrix' tablet. Compressive force, 2 kN; core:coat ratio, 1:1.

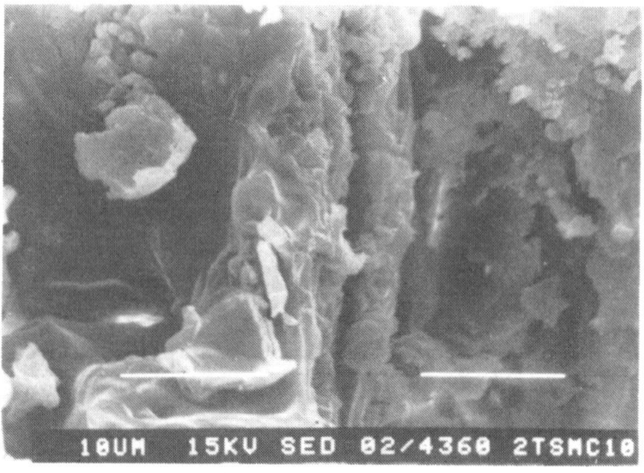

Fig. 4 — Scanning electron micrograph of the tablet surface from a 'microcap' tablet, after dissolution. Compressive force, 10 kN; core:coat ratio, 2:1.

result at 2 kN was very different from that at 5 or 10 kN. In the former the 2:1 ratio tablets released far more rapidly than the 1:1 ratio tablets; about 60% more over a period of 2 h. At 5 and 10 kN the rate of release from both tablet ratios was approximately the same, with the 2:1 ratio tablets reaching the steady rate of release earlier.

At pH 7 (Fig. 6) the 2:1 matrix tablets still show a significantly faster release than does the 1:1 system. The latter system, when prepared under both 5 and 10 kN compressive forces, releases more slowly than either of the two microencapsulated

Table 2 — Amount of drug released from phenobarbitone–poly (DL-lactic acid) tablets

pH	Time (min)	Amount released (mg) for the following compressive forces and systems[a]											
		2kN				5 kN				10 kN			
		A	B	C	D	A	B	C	D	A	B	C	D
2	5	0.0	1.7	1.7	1.7	1.4	1.7	1.7	1.7	1.4	0.0	1.7	1.7
	15	1.4	1.7	3.3	5.0	1.4	1.7	3.3	3.3	1.4	1.7	3.3	3.3
	30	1.4	5.0	8.3	11.6	1.4	3.3	6.6	8.3	1.4	3.3	8.3	8.3
	60	2.8	6.6	13.3	18.2	2.7	5.0	11.6	11.6	2.8	5.0	11.6	11.7
	120	2.8	10.0	18.2	29.8	2.7	8.3	14.9	18.2	4.1	8.3	16.6	19.9
7	30	7.0	9.5	7.3	12.2	7.8	8.7	6.1	11.5	8.2	8.9	3.5	10.7
	120	16.4	19.3	21.4	28.8	16.8	18.6	17.6	26.2	18.2	18.2	14.3	23.7
	180	20.2	24.4	28.6	36.9	21.1	24.0	24.5	32.0	22.6	22.6	19.0	29.5
	240	22.2	28.4	35.3	40.8	24.3	27.3	29.9	37.8	25.8	26.2	23.6	35.3
	300	23.2	31.7	38.4	47.3	26.7	30.6	32.7	43.7	28.2	29.8	25.4	41.1
	360	24.8	37.5	40.0	50.2	28.7	34.9	33.5	48.4	29.9	33.5	26.2	45.9
9	120	19.1	19.2	23.6	33.5	18.7	21.5	24.4	32.9	19.3	20.1	22.2	32.3
	240	27.8	30.3	35.2	50.8	27.8	30.8	34.9	49.7	27.8	28.5	32.2	49.0
	360	34.8	38.2	43.9	62.8	34.9	37.5	42.0	62.0	34.1	34.6	39.3	60.2
	480	41.0	44.6	51.5	73.2	42.3	43.4	47.9	72.6	39.3	41.4	45.2	69.7
	600	46.8	49.8	59.4	83.5	47.8	48.4	53.4	80.4	43.9	46.1	51.2	78.1
	720	52.6	54.3	67.0	92.5	52.1	57.7	58.5	88.5	47.7	50.2	50.4	86.4

[A]Systems and ratios: microcapsules A (1:1), B (2:1); matrices C (1:1), D (2:1).

systems, with the latter showing similar percentage release rates to each other. Over the initial 2 h period as far greater percentage was released from the 'microcap' tablets than in pH 2, but the increase in release from the matrix tablets was by comparison small.

At pH 9 there were significant differences in the percentage released between systems, other than the 2:1 matrices, but the change in preparative compressive forces produced only a small reduction in release.

CONCLUSIONS

Release of the drug from the microcapsules is extremely rapid compared with that from the compressed systems.

The 'microcap' systems showed slower release than the matrices in all three pH values, because release of the drug from the matrix tablets occurs by simple diffusion through the pores existing between poly(DL-lactic acid) plates.

The release from 'microcap' systems is more complicated. First the drug has to dissolve in dissolution fluid which has diffused into the tablets via pores and then between the plates of poly(DL-lactic acid) forming the walls of the microcapsules. This drug solution then has to diffuse out of the tablet via the same route. The effect of compression on the release has more significance in the simple matrix tablets than the 'microcap' systems, because of the above mechanism of release. Higher compressions reduce the size of the pores between the poly(DL-lactic acid) plates, which extends the release.

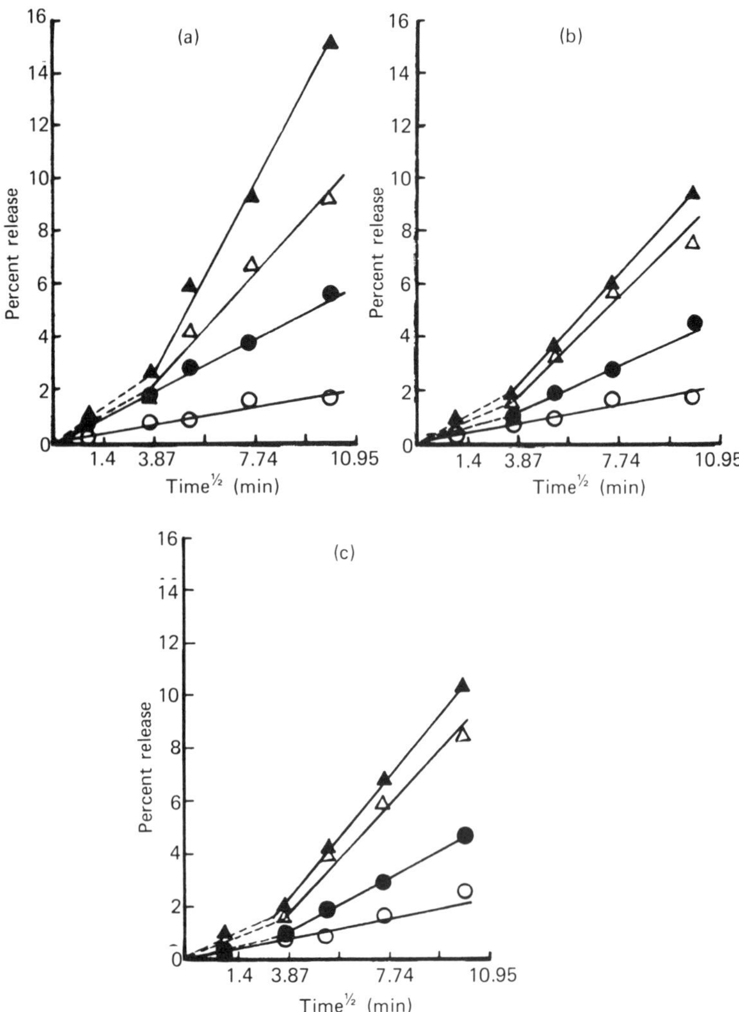

Fig. 5 — 'Higuchi' plot of the release of phenobarbitone from phenobarbitone–DL-PLA tablets. Systems and ratios: microcapsules 1:1; 2:1; matrices 1:1; 2:1; compressive forces (a) 2 kN, (b) 5 kN and (c) 10 kN. Dissolution conditions: Buffer pH 2; stirring rate, 100 rev min^{-1}; t=37°C.

Finally, the drug:polymer ratio plays a substantial role in the amount released. As the drug:polymer ratioo was raised a far more significant difference was noticable in the amount released.

ACKNOWLEDGEMENTS

Miss B. Oraceska thanks Dr M. C. Solomon and DDSA Pharmaceuticals for financial assistance.

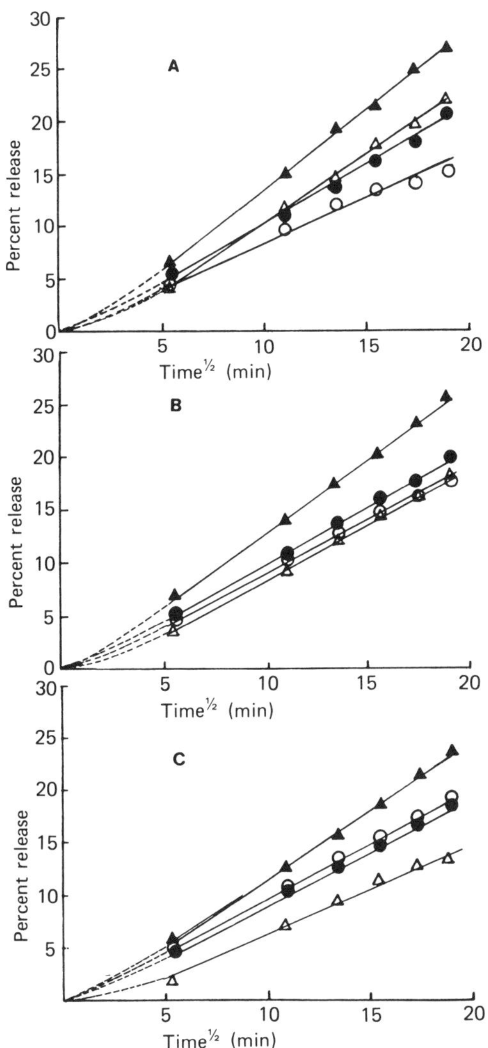

Fig. 6 — 'Higuchi' plot of the release of phenobarbitone from phenobarbitone–DL-PLA tablets. Systems and ratios: microcapsules 1:1; 2:1; matrices 1:1; 2:1; compressive forces (a) 2 kN, (b) 5 kN and (c) 10 kN. Dissolution conditions: Buffer pH 7; stirring rate, 100 rev min^{-1}; t=37°C.

REFERENCES

[1] V. H. Lee and J. R. Robinson, in J. R. Robinson (ed.), *Sustained and Controlled Release Drug Delivery Systems,* Dekker, New York, 1978, p. 123.

[2] W. A. Ritschel, in E. J. Ariens (ed.), *Drug Design,* Vol. IV, Academic Press, New York, 1973, p. 37.

[3] D. A. Wood, in A. T. Florence (ed.), *Materials Used in Pharmaceutical Formulation,* Blackwell, London, 1984, p. 77.

[4] R. K. Kulkarni, K. C. Pani, C. Neuman and F. Leonard, *Arch. Surg.,* **93**, 839 (1966).
[5] S. Yolles, D. J. E. Eldridge and J. H. R. Woodland, *Polym. News,* **1**, 9 (1971).
[6] L. R. Beck, D. R. Cowsar, D. H. Lewis, J. W. Gibson and C. E. Flowers, *Am. J. Obstet. Gynecol.,* **135**, 419 (1979).
[7] L. R. Beck, D. R. Cowsar, D. H. Lewis, R. J. Cosgrove, C. T. Riddel, S. L. Lowry and T. Epperly *Fertil. Steril.,* **31**(5), 545 (1979).
[8] S. Yolles, T. D. Leafe, J. H. R. Woodland and F. J. Meyer, *J. Pharm. Sci.,* **64**(2), 348 (1975).
[9] D. L. Wise, J. D. Greser and G. J. McCormick, *J. Pharm. Pharmacol.,* **31**, 201 (1979).
[10] N. Wakiyama, K. Juni and M. Nakano, *Chem. Pharm. Bull.,* **29**(11), 3363 (1981).
[11] K. Suzuki and J. C. Price, *J. Pharm. Sci.,* **74**(1), 21 (1985).
[12] H. J. Krause, A. Schwarz and P. Rohdewald, *Int. J. Pharm.,* **27**, 145 (1985).
[13] S. Benita, J. P. Benoit, F. Puisieux and C. Thies, *J. Pharm. Sci.,* **73**(12), 1721 (1984).
[14] R. K. Kulkarni, E. G. Moore, A. F. Hegyeli and F. J. Leonard, *Biomed. Mater. Res.,* **5**, 169 (1971).
[15] R. M. Barrer, in J. Crank and G. S. Park (eds.), *Diffusion in Polymers,* Academic Press, London, 1968, p. 165.
[16] A. Schindler, R. Jeffcoat, G. L. Kimmel, C. G. Pitt, M. F. Wall and R. Zweidinger, in J. R. Schaefgen *Contemporary Topics in Polymer Science,* Vol. 2., E. M. Peace and J. R. Schaefgen (eds.), Plenum, New York, 1977, p. 251.
[17] M. D. Coffin, R. Bodmeier, K. T. Chang and J. W. McGinity, *Abstracts 6th Int., Symp. on Microencapsulation Caftat-Dubrovnik, Yugoslavia,* 23–25 September, 1987, Vol. II, p. 31.

Ophthalmic formulation

14

In vitro–in vivo comparison of timolol maleate release from buffered and unbuffered matrices of monoisopropyl ester of poly(vinyl methyl ether–maleic anhydride)

U. Finne, V. Väisänen and **A. Urtti**
Department of Pharmaceutical Technology, University of Kuopio, PO Box 6, 70211 Kuopio, Finland

SUMMARY

Alkyl monoesters of poly(vinyl methyl ether–maleic anhydride) (PVM–MA) are bioerodible acidic polymers that are used to control drug release. In biological fluids with poor buffering capacity, drug release from the polymers and their dissolution are slowed owing to the lower pH on the polymer surface. We studied whether the release of timolol from matrices of monoisopropyl ester of PVM–MA *in vitro* and *in vivo* in rabbits' eyes could be affected by disodium phosphate in the matrices. Addition of disodium phosphate to the matrices doubled the release rate of timolol *in vitro*, but it did not affect the bulk pH of the dissolution medium. On the basis of the timolol concentrations in the tear fluid and in systemic circulation, disodium phosphate seems to accelerate drug release *in vivo* also. Disodium phosphate probably affects the rate of drug release by increasing the microenvironmental pH on the polymer surface.

INTRODUCTION

Bioerodible alkyl monoesters of poly(vinyl methyl ether–maleic anhydride) (PVM–MA) (Fig. 1) can be used to control drug release. Being acidic, ionizable polymers the pH of the disolution medium affects the rate of polymer dissolution [1].

During polymer dissolution, the pH on the polymer surface decreases. This decreases the rate of polymer dissolution. When buffer is added to dissolution

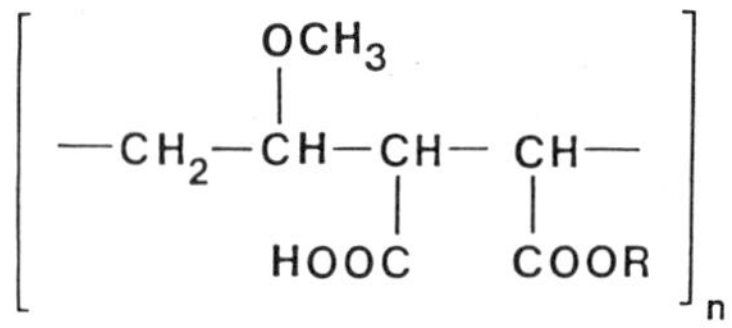

$$\left[-CH_2-\underset{}{\overset{OCH_3}{\overset{|}{C}}}H-\underset{HOOC}{\underset{|}{C}}H-\underset{COOR}{\underset{|}{C}}H- \right]_n$$

Fig. 1 — Structure of PVM–MA.

medium, hydrogen ions are neutralized by the buffer on the surface of the polymer. The buffer concentration thus affects the rates of polymer dissolution and erosion-controlled drug release [1]. In biological fluids with poor buffering capacity, such as tear fluid, dissolution of the polymer is slowed in relation to the rate of solvent penetration into the polymer. Consequently, diffusion and leaching of drug from hydrated polymer increases [2,3].

By adding basic salts to matrices of the isopropyl ester of PVM–MA, the pH on the polymer surface and drug release from the matrices could be increased in dissolution medium with poor buffering capacity [4].

The aim of this study was to find out whether it is possible to affect the dissolution of monoisopropyl ester of PVM–MA and drug release form the polymer *in vivo* in tear fluid by adding basic salts to the matrices. Timolol maleate was used as the drug.

MATERIALS AND METHODS

Materials

Timolol as used as the maleate salt (INTER$_x$ Research Corp., MSDRL, Lawrence, KS, USA). Monoisopropyl ester of PVM–MA was used as 50% isopropanol solution of the polymer (Gantrez® ES-335, GAF Europe, Esher, UK). The radioligand was (–)-^{3}H-CGP-12177 (specific activity, 48.8–53 Ci/mmol, radiochemical purity 99%; Amersham International plc, Buckinghamshire, UK). Mixed-breed pigmented rabbits (1.4–2.8 kg) were used in *in vivo* study. Before the experiments the rabbits were housed singly in standard laboratory conditions: 10 h dark–14 h light cycle, 20–21°C temperature, 40–70% relative air humidity. Food and water were given to the animals *ad libitum*. During the experiments, the rabbits were kept in wooden restraint boxes. Lipoluma™ and Lumasolve™ were purchased from Lumac BV (Schaesberg, The Netherlands).

Preparation of polymer matrices

Matrices of monoisopropyl ester of PVM–MA were prepared by solvent casting. 5 g of 50% isopropanol solution of the polymer were dissolved in 50 ml of acetone-:methanol (1:1) mixture and the solution mixed. 50 mg (0.116 mmol) or 125 mg (0.289 mmol) of timolol were added and the solution was gently mixed for 3 h. The solution was cast on Teflon-coated Petri dishes and allowed to evaporate at room temperature. Circular matrices with diameters of 5 mm (*in vivo* study) or 13 mm (*in vitro* study) were cut with a cork borer and kept in a desiccator until used.

Buffered matrices containing disodium phosphate (2.11 mmol) were prepared as above with the following exception. The salt was first dissolved in a small amount of distilled water, then methanol–polymer mixture and the drug were added. The amount of salt in the matrices was 12.5% or 12.9% (w/w).

Studies of *in vitro* release

The release of timolol from isopropyl PVM–MA matrices used the rotating disk method [5]. The dissolution medium was 100 ml of pH 7.4 2 mM phosphate buffer at 32°C. Ionic strength was adjusted to 0.5 with sodium chloride. Samples of volume 3.0 ml were withdrawn and replaced by dissolution medium. Timolol concentrations were analysed with a UV spectrophotometer at 294 nm and the pH was measured.

Release rates (%/min) were calculated from the best fits of released drug vs. time plots. The slopes (k) of the log(released drug) vs. log(time) plots were calculated from the linear least-squares regression lines. A slope of 0.5 in the log–log plot indicates diffusional, square root of time, dependence and a slope of 1.0 indicates zero-order release kinetics [6]. Times of 50% drug release ($t_{50\%}$) were calculated from the best fits of drug released vs. time plots.

***In vivo* studies**

Matrices of monoisopropyl ester of PVM–MA were carefully applied in the lower conjunctival sac of rabbits. Inserts did not cause any irritation in rabbit eyes. Plasma and tear fluid samples were collected at different times during a period of 8 h. Blood samples were taken from the cannulated ear artery. Plasma was separated by centrifuging (2000 g, 4 min) and kept at −20°C until analysed. Tear fluid samples (1 μl) were collected with microcapillaries at 30, 120, 240 and 480 min after application of the matrices. Tear fluid samples were diluted in 5 ml of phosphate buffer.

Timolol concentration in plasma and tear fluid samples was measured using a modified radioreceptor assay [7]. In the assay, displacement of a β-antagonist, (−)-^{3}H-CGP-12177, from β-receptors of rat reticulocyte membranes by timolol was measured. Rat reticulocyte membranes were obtained as described by Wellstein *et al.* [7].

In a total volume of 300 μl, 50 μl reticulocyte membranes in phosphate buffer (500 μg protein) were incubated for 60 min at 25°C with 50 μl (30 nCi) of (−)-3H-CGP-12177, 180 μl of plasma and 20 μl of 310 mOsm sodium phosphate buffer (pH 7.4). Standard curves were run for each rabbit separately in order to avoid errors due to possible differences in protein binding. To generate the standard curves, blank plasma was used and incubated in the presence of 1–20 nM timolol. For the determination of non-specific binding, incubation in a 10^{-5} M propranolol solution was used.

Timolol concentration in tear fluid samples was measured in the same way, but 200 μl of the diluted tear fluid in phosphate buffer were used instead of 180 μl plasma. After incubation, bound and free radioligand were separated by vacuum filtration through Whatman GF/F glass fibre filters. Filters were washed three times with 10 ml ice-cold 310 mOsm phosphate buffer, dried and counted for retained radioactivity in 5 ml of Lipoluma–Lumasolve–water (10:1:0.2) mixture using Rackbeta 1216 and 1218 liquid scintillation counters (LKB Wallac, Turku, Finland). Counting was continued for 5 min or until 5000 counts. Statistical significance of the differences was tested using Mann–Whitney's *U* test. $p<0.05$ was considered to be a statistically significant difference.

The amount of timolol in the matrices did not affect the relative rate of drug release from matrices of monoisopropyl ester of PVM–MA (Table 1, Fig. 2). The

Table 1 — Release of timolol from buffered and unbuffered matrices of monoisopropyl ester of PVM–MA in 2 mM phosphate buffer solution (pH 7.40) at 32°C

Timolol (mg)	Phosphate buffer (mmol)	k^a	Release rate (%/min)	$t_{50\%}$ (min)	n	pH[b]
50	—	0.90±0.01	0.17±0.01	265.7±10.1	5	6.37
50	2.11	1.16±0.08	0.34±0.02[c]	150.4± 2.8[c]	5	6.33
125	—	0.91±0.01	0.18±0.01	262.4±13.3	6	6.31
125	2.11	0.85±0.01	0.36±0.01[d]	120.2± 4.3[c,d]	6	6.33

Means ± SEM of n experiments are shown.
[a] Slope of log(released timolol) vs. log(time) plot.
[b] pH at the end of the release experiment.
[c,d] $p<0.005$ (Mann–Whitney *U* test). Result was compared with timolol release from unbuffered matrices containing [c] 50 mg or [d] 125 mg of timolol.

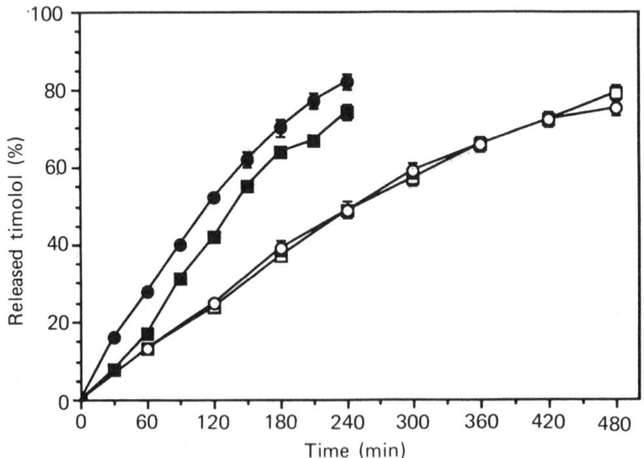

Fig. 2 — Release of timolol (%) from buffered (■, ●) and unbuffered (□,○) matrices of monoisopropyl ester of PVM–MA containing 50 mg (■,□) or 125 mg (●,○) timolol in 2 mM phosphate buffer solution (pH 7.4). Means ± SEM are presented.

matrices did not dissolve completely in 2 mM phosphate buffer solution during the release experiment. The release of timolol from the matrices was close to zero-order kinetics (k=1.0) and differed clearly from diffusional, square root of time, kinetics (k=0.5) (Table 1, Fig. 2). When 2.11 mmol of disodium phosphate were added to the matrices the release rate of timolol was approximately doubled. The phosphate did not affect the bulk pH in the end of experiment (Table 1). Consequently, the faster release rate of timolol from matrices with disodium phosphate is due to the higher pH on the polymer surface. Higher pH increases the rate of polymer dissolution and as a consequence drug release is accelerated.

The peak timolol concentration (7.0±1.5 ng/ml) in plasma occurred at 60 min with the buffered matrices (Fig. 3). After administration of unbuffered matrix a steady state level of 1.0±0.1 ng/ml in plasma was achieved at 3 h (Fig. 3).

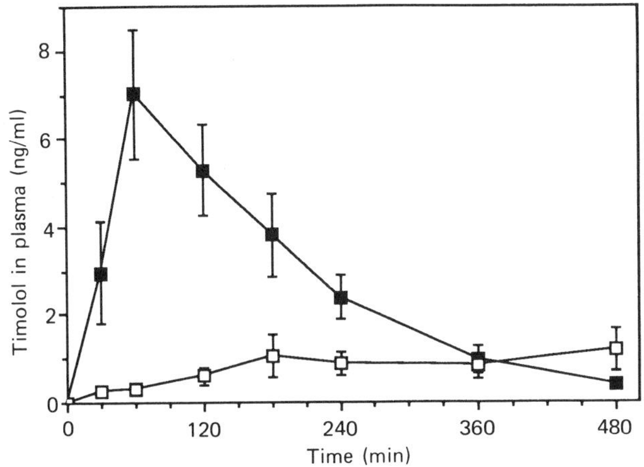

Fig. 3 — Timolol concentration (μg/ml) in plasma after application of one buffered (■) or unbuffered (□) matrix in each eye of a rabbit. Means ± SEM of 5–9 rabbits are shown.

The concentration profiles in tear fluid (Fig. 4) resemble the profiles in plasma (Fig. 3). Compared with unbuffered matrix (c_{max} = 45.2±9.4 μg/ml) administration of timolol in polymer matrix with disodium phosphate resulted in a higher peak (91.5±13.7 μg/ml) in tear fluid (Fig. 4). With the unbuffered matrices, the peak levels of timolol in tear fluid were seen much later than with buffered matrices (Fig. 4).

Timolol concentrations in the tear fluid and plasma suggest that compared with unbuffered matrices timolol is released more rapidly from the isopropyl ester of PVM–MA matrices with disodium phosphate *in vivo*. During the experiment, the buffered matrices also dissolved more rapidly in the tear fluid than the unbuffered matrices.

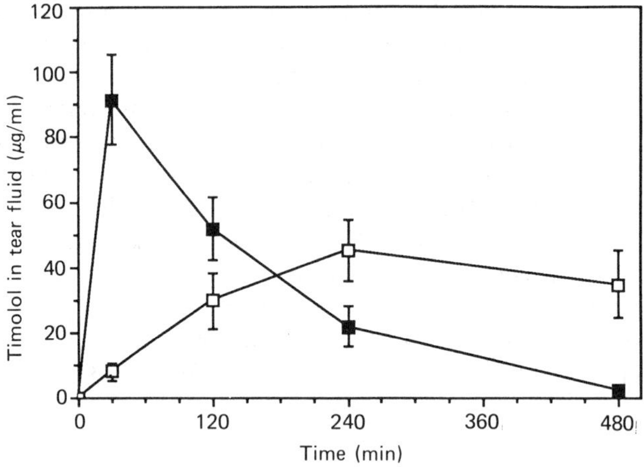

Fig. 4 — Timolol concentration (μg/ml) in tear fluid after application of one buffered (■) or unbuffered (□) matrix in each eye of a rabbit. Means ± SEM of 11–18 eyes are shown.

In vivo results correspond quite well to those of the *in vitro* experiments although the effect of a basic additive seems to be greater *in vivo*. It is possible to increase the dissolution rate of PVM–MA esters in tear fluid by adding disodium phosphate or possibly other basic salts to the matrices. With basic additives it may be possible to modify drug release and polymer dissolution also in the case of other polyacids.

ACKNOWLEDGEMENTS

The polymer Gantrez® ES-335 was a generous gift from GAF (NORDEN) AB (Johanneshov, Sweden). Timolol was a generous gift from $INTER_x$ Research Corp., MSDRL (Lawrence, KS, USA). We are grateful to Mrs Lea Pirskanen for her skilful technical assistance.

REFERENCES

[1] J. Heller, R. W., Baker, R. M. Gale and J. O. Rodin, Controlled release by polymer dissolution I. Partial esters of maleic anhydride copolymers — properties and theory, *J. Appl. Polym. Sci.*, **22**, 1991 (1978).

[2] A. Urtti, Pilocarpine release from matrices of alkyl half-esters of poly(vinyl methyl ether/maleic anhydride), *Int. J. Pharm.*, **26**, 45 (1985).

[3] A. Urtti, L. Salminen and O. Miinalainen, Systemic absorption of ocular pilocarpine is modified by polymer matrices, *Int. J. Pharm.*, **23**, 147 (1985)

[4] U. Finne, K. Kyyrönen and A. Urtti, Buffering of matrix modifies drug release from monoisopropyl ester of PVM/MA, *Proc. Int. Symp. Control. Release Bioact. Mater.*, **15**, 386 (1988).

[5] K. G. Mooney, M. A. Mintun, K. J. Himmelstein and V. J. Stella, Dissolution kinetics of carboxylic acids I: effect of pH under unbuffered conditions, *J. Pharm. Sci.,* **70**, 13 (1981).
[6] J. B. Schwartz, A. P. Simonelli and W. I. Higuchi, Drug release from wax matrices I. Analysis of data with first-order kinetics and with the diffusion-controlled model, *J. Pharm. Sci.,* **57**, 274 (1968).
[7] A. Wellstein, D. Palm, G. Wiemer, M. Schäfer-Korting and E. Mutschler, Simple and reliable radioreceptor assay for beta-adrenoceptor antagonists and active metabolites in native human plasma, *Eur. J. Clin. Pharmacol.,* **27**, 545 (1984).

15

Preparation and evaluation of a sustained release ophthalmic vehicle for dapiprazole

M. F. Saettone, C. Alderigi and **B. Giannaccini**
Department of Pharmaceutical Technology/Biopharmaceutics, University of Pisa, I-56100 Pisa, Italy, and
D. Galli-Angeli
ACRAF SpA, I-60100 Ancona, Italy

SUMMARY

The present investigation is concerned with the development and *in vivo* evaluation of a long-acting ocular vehicle for the α-adrenergic blocking drug dapiprazole (DAP). The approaches tested for prolonging the activity were (a) using the drug base with polygalacturonic acid (PGA) and (b) formulation as a highly viscous hydrogel. The vehicles prepared by applying (singly or in combination) these techniques, and two reference aqueous vehicles containing DAP-HCl, were submitted to a series of biological tests on rabbits (miosis and reversion of mydriasis). When compared with an aqueous solution containing an equivalent amount of DAP-HCl, the polyanionic complex DAP-base–PGA increased significantly some activity parameters (maximal miotic intensity, duration, AUC) of the drug, while the hydrogel vehicle containing DAP-HCl prolonged the apparent absorption and elimination phases of the drug, mainly by virtue of a prolonged ocular retention. The combination of the two approaches, as in the hydrogels containing the DAP–PGA complex, permitted the best control of pharmacological activity parameters, which corresponded to a prolonged-pulse release of the drug. In the miosis test, the AUC values did not show any dose-dependent increase, while this effect was evident in the mydriasis-reversion experiments. The possible mechanism(s), by which the examined techniques may influence the activity parameters and the overall ocular bioavailability of DAP are discussed.

INTRODUCTION

Dapiprazole hydrochloride (DAP-HCl; 5,6,7,8-tetrahydro-3-[2-(4-*o*-tolyl-1-piperazinyl)ethyl;]-*s*-triazole[4,3-*a*]pyridine monohydrochloride) is an α-adrenergic blocking agent, mainly used for the treatment of chronic simple glaucoma in cases where a miotic effect coupled to reduction of intraocular pressure (IOP) is desired [1]. Other therapeutic applications are the induction of pre-operative miosis in specified cases of eye surgery and the reversion of pharmacologically induced mydriasis [2,3]. The drug is clinically used as an aqueous solution, reconstituted prior to use from a freeze-dried formulation Glamidolo®, Angelini).

The topical administration of ophthalmic drugs from aqueous solutions (collyria) is characterized by a poor bioavailability and a short duration of action, as a result of a series of concomitant physiological factors (induced lacrimation, tear turnover, solution drainage etc.) which remove the solution from the eye. These factors have been widely investigated, and several approaches to extending the ocular residence time of topically applied medications have been reported [4]. In the present study two such approaches, namely (a) complexing the basic drug with a polyanionic polymer and (b) increased vehicle viscosity, were applied to the development of a long-acting ocular formulation for DAP. The effect on the biological activity of a series of DAP vehicles was submitted to preliminary *in vivo* tests by performing miosis and reversion of tropicamide-induced mydriasis tests in rabbits.

EXPERIMENTAL

Materials

Dapiprazole base, DAP-B (melting point, 163–164°C), and hydrochloride, DAP-HCL (melting point, 192–193°C), were purified samples supplied by Acraf SpA (Ancona); high molecular weight hydroxypropylcellulose, HPC (Klucel HF, Hercules Inc., Wilmington, DE), and polyglacturonic acid, PGA (4.89 mEq/g, Prion Chemicals, Milano), were commercial samples, used without prior purification. Benzalkonium chloride, USP grade (BZ), was purchased from Carlo Erba SpA; Nylon 6 (Capran 77C, thickness 27±0.3 μm) was obtained from Allied Chemical Corp., Morristown, NJ.

Vehicles

The DAP-B–PGA ionic complex was prepared by adding portionwise, at room temperature, 0.68 g PGA to a stirred solution of FDAP-B (1.0 g) in methanol (50 ml). The solvent was then evaporated to give a highly water soluble creamy white powder, containing 59.52% DAP-B. The pH of a 1.68% w/v solution of the complex (corresponding to 1.0% DAP-B) was 5.4.

The composition of all DAP vehicles is shown in Table 1.

Gel vehicles 5–8 were prepared by adding a water solution of DAP-HCl or PGA complex to a preformed HPC gel containing BZ as the preservative. As an example, the preparation of vehicle 5 is described. A solution of the ionic complex DAP-B–PGA (0.84 g) in water (35 ml) was slowly added, while stirring, to a gel prepared by hydrating overnight 4.5 g HPC in water (60 ml) containing benzalkonium chloride (0.01 g). The mixture was then brought to the final weight, and was stored at 5°C until used.

Table 1 — Composition of dapiprazole vehicles

	Composition of the vehicles							
	1	2	3	4	5	6	7	8
DAP-HCl	0.5	1.0					0.5	1.0
DAP-B–PGA			0.84_a	1.68^b	0.84_a	1.68^b		
HPC					4.5	4.5	4.5	4.5

All vehicles contained water, q.s. to 100 ml, and 0.01% w/v BZ.
[a]Equivalent to 0.5% DAP-B.
[b]Equivalent to 1.0% DAP-B.

***In vitro* release tests**

These tests were performed by measuring the rate of dapiprazole release from gel vehicles 6 and 8 to an aqueous sink, through a non-porous membrane. For this purpose, a thin nylon membrane, which had been preconditioned by extraction with ethanol (1 h at 60°C) and overnight hydration in distilled water at room temperature, was positioned between the receiving (5 ml) and the donating (4 ml) compartment of a glass 'GH' flow-through diffusion cell [5], thermostated at 30°C. At $t=0$ the vehicle was introduced into the upper section of the cell, and the stirred receiving solution (0.01 M HCl) was periodically sampled and analysed spectrophotometrically for DAP-HCl (234 nm), using an appropriate calibration curve. The withdrawn samples were immediately replaced with equal amounts of prewarmed receiving solution.

Biological tests

(a) Miotic activity tests were carried out on non-anaesthetized male albino rabbits weighing 2.5–3.0 kg, using a standard procedure [6]. The vehicle dose, which was applied into the lower conjunctival sac of one eye, was in all cases 50 µl; each vehicle was tested on six animals.

(b) Mydriasis reversion tests were performed on vehicles 1, 5 and 6, using at least six rabbits for each vehicle. For these experiments both eyes of the rabbits were pretreated with 10 µl of a 1.0% commercial solution of tropicamide (Visumidriatic, Merck Sharp & Dohme). After reaching the peak mydriatic effect (c. 25 min), the vehicle under study (50 µl) was applied into the lower conjunctival sac of one eye, and the measurement of the pupillary diameter was performed as indicated previously. The results were expressed as differences in diameter (mm) between the eye treated with tropicamide alone and the eye which had received the DAP vehicle.

RESULTS

In vitro release

These tests had essentially the purpose of providing information on the extent of DAP binding in the PGA ionic complex and on the influence of complexation by

PGA on DAP release from the vehicles. The study was carried out on gel vehicles 6 and 8, containing an equivalent amount of DAP respectively as PGA complex and as hydrochloride. In both cases DAP was released with zero-order kinetics over a period of 36 h; release from vehicle 6, containing the PGA complex, was much slower with respect to vehicle 8, containing the hydrochloride: the slopes of the release plots were 4.83×10^{-3} (K') for vehicle 6, and 2.19×10^{-2} (K) for vehicle 8. As demonstrated in a previous paper for a similar case [7], the ratio of the two slopes, K'/K, is equal to C_f/C_i, where C_i is the total amount of drug in the diffusing medium and C_f is the concentration of 'free' drug, i.e. in equilibrium with drug bound by the PGA complex. A simple calculation shows that in vehicle 6 only 22% of the total amount of drug was in free diffusible form. This value is to be considered indicative, and is based on some simplifying assumptions, the main one of which is that no binding takes place in either vehicle between HPC, the gel-forming agent and dapiprazole.

***In vivo* data: miotic activity**

The results of the miotic activity tests on rabbits carried out with the eight vehicles under investigation are summarized in Table 2

Table 2 — Summary of the miotic activity parameters of the DAP vehicles

Vehicle	Peak time (min)	I_{max} (mm)	Duration (min)	AUC (cm^2) ($\pm$95% CL)	$K'\times1000$ (min^{-1})[a]
1	30	1.87	150	28 (13)	13.7
2	30	1.75	180	33 (9)	13.0
3	120	2.50	290	102 (7)	12.6
4	120	2.50	310	93 (10)	14.1
5	60	2.10	370	86 (14)	3.5
6	60	2.40	380	100 (19)	4.0
7	90	1.60	330	70 (24)	3.2
8	85	2.00	350	98 (14)	2.6

[a]First-order rate constant for elimination, determined from the terminal slopes of the lines of the log (change in pupillary diameter) vs. time plots.

Effect of the applied dose

The preparations listed in Table 2 can be divided into four couples (1–2, 3–4, 5–6, 7–8), in each of which the drug was present at two concentrations, corresponding to 0.5% and 1.0% DAP. An inspection of the data shows that, within each couple, a 100% increased concentration resulted in very little or no increase of the activity parameters. Even if in some cases slightly increased I_{max} (vehicle 6 vs. 5, or vehicle 8 vs. 7) or duration (vehicle 2 vs. 1, or vehicle 8 vs. 7) values were apparent, in no case were the AUC values of each couple of preparations statistically different.

Effect of complexation of DAP-B by PGA

This effect is evidenced by a comparison of the activity data within each one of two vehicle couples, 1–3 and 2–4. In each couple the vehicles contained an equivalent amount of drug (0.5% or 1.0%), but in a different form (HCl or PGA complex). Within each couple, the presence of the PGA complex resulted in a significant (c. 3 times) increase in bioavailability, associated with an increase in duration and intensity of activity. Complexation of DAP-B by PGA had little effect on the apparent (Newtonian) viscosities of the vehicles (which were 1.4 and 1.7 mPa s for vehicles 3 and 4, vs. c. mPa 1.0 s for vehicles 1 and 2, at 30°C) so that a possible influence of viscosity effects on the ocular retention, and hence on the activity of the PGA complex, should be ruled out. The apparent elimination kinetics of vehicles 1–4 (reflected by the K' values in Table 2), which were in the same range as those of vehicles 1 and 2, suggests a relatively short pre-ocular retention. This is in contrast with the high AUC values of the vehicles.

Effect of gelling by HPC

This effect can best be appraised by comparing the activity parameters within each of two groups of vehicles 1–3–5–7 (0.5% DAP) or 2–4–6–8 (1.0% DAP). The reported data show that, within the first group, the presence of HPC (and the associated great increase of vehicle viscosity) had a positive effect on bioavailability (2.5×) when the drug was present as the hydrochloride (vehicle 7 vs. 1). A similar AUC increase was not apparent when the drug was present in the gels as the PGA complex (vehicle 5 vs. 3). In other words, addition of the gel-forming cellulose derivative was apparently unable to increase the AUC values displayed by the liquid vehicles containing the PGA salt. Similar considerations apply to the other group of vehicles (1.0% DAP). The gel vehicles, however, appeared to exert some control on DAP release and absorption, as indicated by an increased duration of activity (cf. for example vehicles 7 and 8 vs. 1 and 2 respectively) and by consistently lower K' values, corresponding to a prolongation of the apparent absorption and elimination phases of the drug in the eye.

***In vivo* reversion of mydriasis**

Administration of 0.1 mg tropicamide to both eyes of the rabbits produced an intense mydriatic effect, which began slowly to decline after 90 min, but was still very evident (c. 70% of the peak intensity) after 7 h. The results of tests in which the dapiprazole vehicles 1 (reference), 5 and 6 were applied to one of the dilated eyes are illustrated in Fig. 1, where the area corresponding to the reversion effect vs. time of each vehicle are outlined. In Fig. 1, the data are expressed as differences in pupillary diameter, $\Delta\phi$, between the DAP-treated and the dilated, contralateral eye, vs. time. As shown, vehicle 1 produced a reversion of short duration, while the effect of an equivalent dose of DAP (as PGA complex) administered in the gel vehicle 5 was significantly greater, for both intensity and duration, and was still evident after 7 h. Contrary to the miosis experiments, in these tests a 2-fold increase of the administered drug dose (vehicle 6 vs. 5) produced a significantly increased biological response. The relative AUC values for vehicles 1, 5 and 6 (calculated at 2 h, corresponding to the end of the

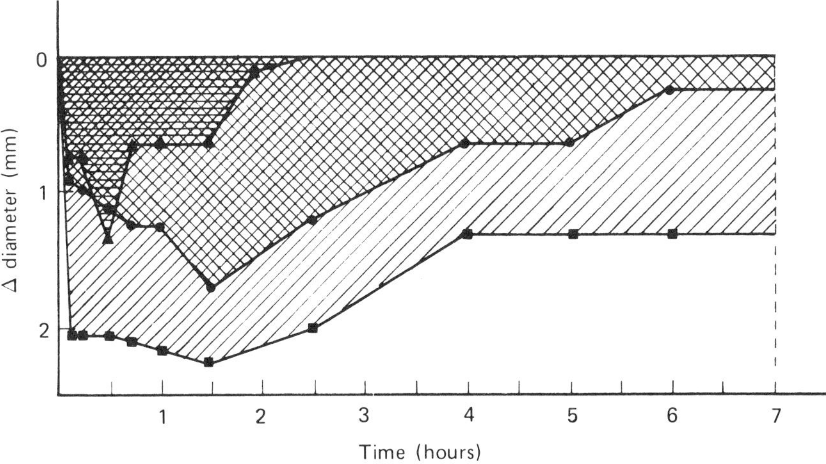

Fig. 1 — Effect of DAP vehicles 1 (▲), 5 (●) and 6 (■) on reversal of tropicamide-induced mydriasis.

effect of vehicle 1) were 1, 1.94 and 3.2. The corresponding relative AUC values at the end of the experiment (7 h) were 1.0, 4.5 and 8.5, respectively.

DISCUSSION

The approaches to enhance and/or prolong the ocular activity of DAP evaluated in the present study, although not unprecedented, differ in some respects from previous literature examples. Salification of pilocarpine with alginic acid [8], with poly(acrylic acid–lauryl methacrylate) [9], with poly(acrylic acid) [10, 11], etc. has been reported to prolong the activity of the drug when the salts were administered in a solid dosage from (insert) [8,10] or when the complex itself was insoluble in water [9]. The 'hydrogel' approach, on the other hand, has been applied to various ophthalmic drugs, and 3–5-fold increases in penetration and activity have been reported. The combined effect of the two techniques has apparently never been investigated, with the possible exception of an example mentioned in the patent literature, (a poly(acrylic acid) hydrogel partially neutralized by pilocarpine base [11]).

The PGA salt of DAP has shown pharmacological results (peak timer shifted to a later time, increased I_{max}) corresponding to an increased contact time [12]. PGA consists of linear chains of D-galacturonic acid units (pyranose form), joined in α(1–4)-glycosidic linkages, with a molecular weight ranging from 25×10^3 to 100×10^3. It formed a soluble salt or polyanionic complex with the sparingly soluble DAP-B, from which the bound drug was released *in vitro* at a slow rate. The remarkable (more than 3-fold) AUC increases produced by the DAP-B–PGA vehicles, whose viscosity was low, cannot be rationalized in terms of a viscosity-induced reduction of the ocular drainage rate. Furthermore, as pointed out by Lee and Robinson [4], only moderate increases in ocular bioavailability may be observed as a result of a significant, viscosity-induced reductions of solution drainage, partly on account of conjunctival absorption. The apparent rate constants for elimination of the DAP-B–PGA liquid vehicles, which are in the same range as those of the DAP-HCl solutions, would also point to a short ocular retention of the former vehicles. The strong and somewhat delayed pulse of miotic activity observed with the DAP-B–PGA liquid vehicles might tentatively be explained in terms of adhesion of the polymer salt to the mucin layer at the corneal surface, leading to a temporary retention and to an improved drug penetration. There are sufficient structural affinities between PGA and the polysaccharide portion of mucin to justify this assumption, and a large amount of evidence has been gathered on the capacity of some polyanionic polymers to interact with and to adhere to the mucin layer of conjunctival tissues [13].

While the PGA liquid vehicles proved capable of greatly enhancing the ocular bioavailability of DAP, their enhanced-pulse delivery might not be quite satisfactory for therapeutic purposes. High values of the peak miotic intensity, corresponding to high aqueous humour levels of the drug, are not desirable since they might intensify dose-related side effects of the drug [14]. On the other hand, the hydrogel vehicles containing DAP-HCl showed activity parameters corresponding to a prolonged retention, as indicated in particular by the low values of the elimination rate constants, reflecting a sustained absorption, distribution and elimination of the drug [15]. It is speculated that the combination of the two techniques might provide an optimization of the activity. The resulting vehicles (5 and 6) appeared indeed to provide the best activity characteristics (long duration, satisfactory but not excessive peak miotic intensity), corresponding to a prolonged-pulse delivery of the drug. The highly viscous gel matrix apparently acted by assisting the ocular retention of the polyanionic complex, thus providing the best conditions for a prolonged release.

The same gel vehicles (5 and 6) also showed remarkably prolonged activity characteristics in the mydriasis reversion tests. In these experiments, contrary to the miosis tests, significant dose-dependent effects could be observed. This phenomenon might be attributed to the more complex pharmacological situation existing in the reversal tests, where a competitive interaction might occur between the mydriatic and the miotic agent for the corresponding receptors.

In conclusion, the remarkable influence on DAP activity exerted by the low-viscosity PGA vehicles is an issue deserving further attention, in view of the possible implication of a muco-adhesive mechanism. A closer study of the potential interactive properties of polyuronic acids and of their drug salts with the precorneal mucin might lead to a better understanding of the bioadhesive properties of these and other similar anionic polymeric materials, and of their influence on ocular drug bioavailability.

REFERENCES

[1] *Annnu. Drug Data Rep.*, **4**, 65 (1982).

[2] B. Silvestrini, L. Bonomi, R. Lisciani, S. Perfetti, R. Bellucci, F. Massa and A. Baldini, *Arzneim.-Forsch.*, **32**, 678 (1982).

[3] B. Brogliatti, T. Rolle, M. Messelod and B. Boles-Caarenini, *Glaucoma (USA),* **6**, 110 (1985).
[4] V. H. L. Lee and J. R. Robinson, *J. Ocul. Pharmacol.,* **2**, 67 (1986).
[5] C. L. Gummer, R. S. Hinz and H. I. Maibach, *Int. J. Pharm.,* **40**, 101 (1987).
[6] M. F. Saettone, B. Giannaccini, A. Guiducci and P. Savigni, *Int. J. Pharm.,* **31**, 261 (1986).
[7] F. Bottyari, F. Di Colo, E. Nannipieri, M. F. Saettone and M. F. Serafini, *J. Pharm. Sci.*, **64**, 946 (1975).
[8] S. P. Loucas and H. M. Haddad, *Metab. Ophthalmol.,* **1**, 27 (1976).
[9] U. Ticho, M. Blumenthal, S. Zonis, A. Gal, I. Blank and Z. W. Mazor, *Ann. Ophthalmol.,* **11**, 555 (1979).
[10] M. F. Saettone, B. Giannaccini, P. Chetoni, G. Galli and E. Chiellini, *J. Pharm. Pharmacol.*, **36**, 229 (1984).
[11] R. D. Schoenwald and R. E. Roehrs, *US Patent 4,2711,143,* 2 June, 1981.
[12] J. W. Sieg and J. R. Robinson, *J. Pharm. Sci.,* **66**, 1222 (1977).
[13] H. W. Hui and J. R. Robinson, *Int. J. Pharm.,* **26**, 203 (1985).
[14] L. Salminen, A. Urtti, h. Kujari and M. Juslin, *Grafe's Arch. Clin. Exp. Ophthalmol.,* **221**, 96 (1983).
[15] S. S. Chrai and J. R. Robinson, *J. Pharm. Sci.,* **63**, 1218 (1974).

Implants

16

Release kinetics of tobramycin sulphate from polymethylmethacrylate implants

D. H. Robinson and **S. Sampath**
Department of Pharmaceutical Sciences, University of Nebraska Medical Center, Omaha, NE 68105 USA

SUMMARY

The effects of various formulation factors on the *in vitro* release characteristics of spherical polymethylmethacrylate implants were studied. Physical and mathematical models were proposed to describe the *in vitro* release profiles. The *in vitro* release data could be described by a bi-exponential equation of the following type: fraction of tobramycin remaining in the implant at time $t = Ae^{-\alpha t} + Be^{-\beta t}$, where α, and β represent the rate constants for the initial rapid and subsequent slow phases of release. The influence of drug loading, volume of dissolution medium, implant size and type of cement and the incorporation of water-soluble additives on the release profiles and α and β rate constants is described.

INTRODUCTION

Antibiotic-impregnated polymethylmethacrylate (PMMA) bone cement has been used for localized drug delivery in osteomyelitis since 1970 [1–3]. More recently, antibiotic–bone cement composites have been fabricated as spherical, non-biodegradable implants [4]. The primary advantage of localized drug delivery with implants is that relatively high local tissue antibiotic concentrations are obtained without corresponding high serum levels and associated toxicity. Implants containing various antibiotics have been extemporaneously prepared for clinical use. However, many aspects regarding the preparation and release characteristics of these implants have not been clearly defined.

The purpose of this study was to adopt a systematic approach to optimize formulation and to characterize the properties of tobramycin–PMMA implants.

Tobramycin was selected as it is active against both Gram-positive and Gram-negative bacteria, including gentamicin-resistant *Pseudomonas*. The specific aims of the study were

(1) to study the *in vitro* and *in vivo* release characteristics of tobramycin sulphate from the PMMA implant delivery system, and
(2) to develop physical and mathematical models which describe the drug release profiles *in vitro* and account for the observed changes in rate and extent of release between formulations.

THEORETICAL

Mathematical model

Guy *et al.* [5] derived an equation for the diffusion-controlled release of a drug from a sphere, radius r, by applying the three-dimensional form of Fick's second law of diffusion after transformation to spherical coordinates. This equation can be rearranged as:

$$1-\frac{M_t}{M_\infty}=\frac{6}{\pi^2}\sum_{n=1}^{\infty}\frac{1}{n^2}\exp(-n^2\pi^2\tau) \tag{1}$$

The term $1-M_t/M_\infty$ represents the fraction of drug remaining unreleased while τ is a function of the diffusion constant, D, as defined by the equation $\tau=Dt/r^2$. Therefore, the decline in the fraction of drug remaining (fraction released) can be described by a multiexponential equation of the type:

$$\text{fraction of drug remaining}=A\mathrm{e}^{-\alpha t}+B\mathrm{e}^{-\beta t}+\ldots \tag{2}$$

Since r is constant for a non-biodegradable carrier such as PMMA, the slopes α, β, etc., should reflect changes in the diffusion coefficient D, and therefore differences in porosity, between formulations. The first-order drug release rate constants can be calculated from the slopes of the α and β phases of the release profile.

Physical model

Since PMMA is non-biodegradable and resistant to erosion, the dimensions of the spherical implant will not change for the duration of the release process. It was proposed that a biphasic release profile would be observed. An initial, relatively rapid release phase would be observed as a result of the diffusion and dissolution of drug on, or near, the surface of the implant. A second, more prolonged release phase would then follow because of the slow diffusion of the drug from within the PMMA implant matrix. Further, the rate and extent of drug release from the implant during the second prolonged phase could be significantly altered using formulation additives which modify the porosity of the PMMA implant matrix.

METHODS

Materials

Tobramycin sulphate (Nebcin®, lot number 1CE30C) was donated by Eli Lilly Co., Indianapolis, IN. Palacos® cement (lot number 608/7796) was donated by Richards Medical, Memphis, TN. Simplex® cement (lot number HR203-4) and Zimmer Low Viscosity® cement (lot number 51738000) were donated by Howmedica, New York, NY, and Zimmer, Warsaw, IN, respectively. Disodium phosphate (lot number 0201ML) and polyethylene glycols PEG 3400 (lot number 01224MP) and PEG 400 (lot number 97901DM) were purchased from Aldrich Chemical Co. Inc., Milwaukee, WS. Potassium dihydrogen phosphate (lot number 7100KBS) and methylene chloride (lot number 4881KBCL) were obtained from Mallinckrodt Inc., St. Louis, MO. *o*-Phthaldialdehyde reagent solution (lot number 58F-5985) and isopropanol (lot number 78F-6185) were purchased from Sigma Chemical Co., St. Louis, MO. Lactose was obtained from Amend Drugs and Chemical Co., Irvington, CO.

Preparation of implants

Spherical PMMA implants containing tobramycin sulphate were prepared using a Teflon-coated stainless steel mould. All chemicals and equipment were cooled at 4°C before use to retard polymerization rate and to facilitate easier preparation of the implants. Known quantities of tobramycin sulphate were mixed with solid PMMA using geometric dilution, and then the liquid monomer was added to initiate polymerization. Where applicable, solid additives (lactose and PEG 3400) were added to the solid PMMA before the addition of monomer while the liquid additive PEG 400 was added after the addition of monomer. Immediately after mixing thoroughly, the liquid dispersion was injected into the lubricated mould. After solidifying, the implants were removed, allowed to dry at room temperature for 24 h, and then stored for at least four days before testing to ensure loss of residual monomer and completion of polymerization. Initial studies indicated that polymerized methylmethacrylate bone cement attained constant weight after about 24 h.

Weight variation and diameter variation

The mean weight and standard deviation of ten samples from each batch were determined for weight variation. Variation in diameter of beads was determined using a micrometer. The mean diameter (n=6) and the standard deviation were calculated for each batch.

Assay of drug content

Three implants from each batch were assayed separately for tobramycin sulphate content by dissolving the PMMA in 45 ml of dichloromethane and extracting the tobramycin sulphate five times with 5 ml of deionized distilled water. The aqueous extracts were bulked and the volumes adjusted to 50 ml.

Analysis of tobramycin sulphate

Tobramycin sulphate was determined spectrophotometrically using a derivatization procedure [6]. A 0.5–1 ml aliquot of the extracted solution was mixed with 1 ml of *o*-phthaldialdehyde reagent solution followed by addition of 1.5 ml of isopropanol to prevent precipitation. The volume was adjusted to 5 ml with distilled water and the absorbance was determined after 45 min on a Beckman DU-7 spectrophotometer at the maxima of 333 nm. The concentrations were obtained from a calibration curve of *o*-phthaldialdehyde-derivatized tobramycin. The assay had a coefficient of variation of less than 3% and a detection limit of 0.5 μg/ml.

***In vitro* dissolution**

Dissolution kinetics was studied under sink conditions by placing one implant in varying volumes (usually 100 ml) of phosphate buffer pH 7.4, while agitating in a horizontally shaking water bath (50±1 rev/min) at 37±1°C. Samples were withdrawn at varying time intervals for a duration of 21 days (an estimate of the expected duration of clinical use) and the amount of tobramycin sulphate released was determined spectrophotometrically. Equal volumes of fresh medium were added to replace aliquots removed for assay and the amount of drug release was corrected for dilution. Triplicate measurements were performed for each batch of implants prepared.

Formulation factors

The influence of the following formulation factors on the release of tobramycin sulphate from PMMA carrier was studied:

(1) Drug loading: the drug-to-carrier ratio (tobramycin sulphate:PMMA). Drug:-carrier ratios (dry weight) of 1:33 (clinically used), 1:20, 1:10, and 1:5 were used.
(2) Influence of water-soluble formulation additives: PEG 400, PEG 3400 and lactose.
(3) Type of commercial PMMA bone cement: the cements studied were Simplex, Zimmer and Palacos.
(4) Effect of dissolution volume: 100 ml, 10 ml, 5 ml, and 2 ml.
(5) Effect of size: implants in two sizes of 2.9 mm and 6.2 mm diameter were studied.

Palacos bone cement was used for studies in (1), (2), (4) and (5) above. A drug-to-carrier ratio of 1:10 was used for studies in (2)–(5). Implants of diameter 6.2 mm were used in studies (1)–(4).

***In vivo* release**

The rabbit osteomyelitic model described by Norden [7] was used to assess *in vivo* release of tobramycin sulphate from PMMA implants. The implants contained a mean tobramycin sulphate content of 6.1 mg per implant (which corresponds to almost double the drug loading used clinically). Osteomyelitis was induced in the tibia of nine New Zealand rabbits using *Pseudomonas aeruginosa*. One implant was surgically placed immediately adjacent to the tibia infection site in each rabbit 23 days post-infection. Implants were then surgically removed from each of three rabbits 1, 3 and 7 days after implantation and the amount of drug remaining unreleased determined spectrophotometrically after extraction as described above.

Scanning electron microscopy

A Philips model 515 scanning electron microscope was used to study the changes in surface topography of implants both before and after *in vitro* dissolution and after implementation in the rabbit.

Data analysis

Non-linear regression analysis of the *in vitro* release data was performed using the JANA multiexponential curve stripping computer program. The mono-, bi- and triexponential fits were generated. Statistical analysis of computer generated parameters was performed using ANOVA and Student's *t* test. Fisher's LSD was used for the multiple comparison of statistically significant groups.

RESULTS AND DISCUSSION

The mean diameters of the large and small beads were 6.2 mm and 2.9 mm respectively with the coefficients of variation less than 2% within a batch. Mean masses of the batches of the larger beads ranged from 151.8 to 162.5 mg and the smaller beads had a mean mass of 19.9 mg. In no instance was the coefficient of variation for within batch variation greater than 3%.

The correlation coefficients generated for mono-, bi- and triexponential fits obtained by non-linear regression analyses are summarized in Table 1. Wilson *et al.* [8] reported that the rate of tobramycin release from Simplex PMMA beads could be fitted to monoexponential and power functions; however, they obtained r^2 values<0.9 for both fits. Our results show that, although the monoexponential fit is poor, both biexponential and triexponential fits provided r^2 values>0.9. Since the biexponential relationship in equation (2) is proposed to fit our physical model, this approach was adopted in analysis of computer fits to release data. The rate constants, α and β, represent an initial, rapid surface release and a prolonged matrix diffusion-controlled release respectively.

Several investigators have reported that palacos PMMA cement releases antibiotics at higher concentrations over more prolonged periods than other commercially available cements [9–11]; others have suggested that there are no significant differences [12]. Von Frauhofer *et al.* [13] noted that the rates of leaching of tobramycin from three commercial brands of cement were similar, but the initial amount of drug released differed. Our studies indicated that statistical comparison of the rate constants obtained using Palacos, Simplex and Zimmer cements (at similar levels of drug loading) revealed no significant differences ($p>0.1$). Also all three cements showed similar extents of release for the duration of study. Palacos bone cement was used for all subsequent studies.

Table 2 summarizes the effect of various formulation factors on the fast and slow phase rate constants influence of various formulation factors. For all subsequent discussion, the criterion for statistical significance was $p<0.1$.

Table 1 — Determination coefficients for the fitting of *in vitro* data to multiexponential equations

Formulation factor	Tobramycin[a] content (mg) (mean±SD)	R^2 values for exponential fits		
		Mono	Bi	Tri
Effect of drug loading				
1:33	2.9 ±0.009	0.4565	0.9432	0.9810
1:20	4.73±0.269	0.5052	0.9650	0.9908
1:10	9.41±0.423	0.6430	0.9731	0.9860
1:5	17.95±0.069	0.7796	0.9856	0.9927
Effect of additives				
10% PEG 400	9.13±0.139	0.9064	0.9944	0.9974
20% PEG 400	9.34±0.386	0.9295	0.9951	0.9980
30% PEG 400	10.21±0.190	0.6585	0.9841	0.9793
10% PEG 3400	8.21±0.294	0.8222	0.9799	0.9883
10% Lactose	8.72±0.322	0.6667	0.9796	0.9916
Effect of size				
2.9 mm diameter	1.49±0.01	0.2225	0.9103	0.9782
Effect of type of PMMA bone cement				
Zimmer	10.38±0.446	0.7560	0.9445	0.9790
Simplex	10.31±0.218	0.6277	0.9552	0.9902

[a]Drug content determined by spectrophotometric analysis.

Fig. 1 and Table 2 summarize the effect of drug loading on the release profiles of tobramycin. During the rapid initial phase, release rates were all of the same order of magnitude although, at the highest drug loading (17.9 mg/implant), differences were observed in the extent of release. Similarly for the slow phase, significant differences in the β rate constant occurred only at the highest drug loading. At the tobramycin sulphate:PMMA ratio commonly used clinically, i.e. 1:33, the release is incomplete (18–20%) with essentially no drug released after three days. Our studies confirmed the work of Goodell *et al.* [14], who found that over a period of 12 weeks less than 20% of the theoretically available tobramycin was released from beads prepared using a ratio of 1:33 of drug to polymer (dry weight. Studies by Wilson *et al.* also showed that substantial amounts of tobramycin remain in the beads after 28 days.

Our studies indicated that the inclusion of water-soluble additives could alter both the rate and extent of tobramycin release from Palacos PMMA. The three additives PEG 3400, PEG 400 and lactose significantly affected the slower diffusion phase of the matrix (Fig. 2 and Table 2).

Law *et al.* [15] determined the diffusion coefficient for benzyl penicillin in thin films of Palacos, Simplex and CMW cements assuming that antibiotic transport can be described by Fick's law using a finite difference approximation to quantify

Table 2 — Effect of formulation factors on computer–generated fast (α) and slow (β) phase rate constants

Formulation factor	α (h^{-1}) (mean±SD)	β (h^{-1}) (mean±SD)
Effect of drug loading		
1:33	$3.47\times10^{-1}\pm1.11\times10^{-1}$	$1.29\times10^{-4}\pm1.38\times10^{-5}$
1:20	$1.93\times10^{-1}\pm1.01\times10^{-1}$	$1.67\times10^{-4}\pm1.92\times10^{-5}$
1:10	$9.65\times10^{-2}\pm6.63\times10^{-3}$	$1.82\times10^{-4}\pm3.10\times10^{-5}$
1:5	$1.01\times10^{-1}\pm1.65\times10^{-2}$	$1.17\times10^{-3}\pm6.32\times10^{-4}$
Effect of implant size		
6.2 mm	$9.65\times10^{-2}\pm6.63\times10^{-3}$	$1.82\times10^{-4}\pm3.10\times10^{-5}$
2.9 mm	$5.35\times10^{-1}\pm3.63\times10^{-1}$	$1.19\times10^{-3}\pm1.03\times10^{-4}$
Effect of type of cement		
Palacos	$9.65\times10^{-2}\pm6.63\times10^{-3}$	$1.82\times10^{-4}\pm3.10\times10^{-5}$
Zimmer	$1.85\times10^{-1}\pm1.30\times10^{-1}$	$3.17\times10^{-4}\pm9.90\times10^{-5}$
Simplex	$1.75\times10^{-1}\pm1.14\times10^{-1}$	$1.83\times10^{-4}\pm8.23\times10^{-5}$
Effect of soluble additives (10%)		
Control[a]	$9.65\times10^{-2}\pm6.63\times10^{-3}$	$1.82\times10^{-4}\pm3.10\times10^{-5}$
PEG 400	$7.29\times10^{-2}\pm4.02\times10^{-2}$	$3.02\times10^{-4}\pm3.51\times10^{-6}$
PEG 3400	$1.41\times10^{-2}\pm1.74\times10^{-2}$	$9.01\times10^{-4}\pm8.70\times10^{-5}$
Lactose	$9.67\times10^{-2}\pm5.01\times10^{-3}$	$6.30\times10^{-4}\pm3.78\times10^{-5}$
Effect of increasing levels of PEG 400		
Control[a]	$9.65\times10^{-2}\pm6.63\times10^{-4}$	$1.82\times10^{-4}\pm3.10\times10^{-5}$
10%	$7.29\times10^{-2}\pm4.02\times10^{-2}$	$3.02\times10^{-4}\pm3.51\times10^{-6}$
20%	$3.52\times10^{-1}\pm2.64\times10^{-1}$	$8.51\times10^{-3}\pm1.50\times10^{-3}$
30%	$1.94\times10^{-1}\pm3.20\times10^{-2}$	$8.38\times10^{-3}\pm9.07\times10^{-3}$

[a]No additives.

transient non-steady-state behaviour. These investigators found that the diffusion coefficient was increased in the presence of additives and proposed that the finite difference approach could be applied to determine release of antibiotic from preloaded PMMA beads. Dittgen and Stahlkopf [16] showed that incorporation of amino acids of varying solubilities also affected release of chloramphenicol from polymethacrylic implants. Our studies indicated that, while the presence of lactose and PEG 3400 increased the extent of release to about 50%, PEG 400 had a much more pronounced effect, increasing the extent of release to about 85% after three weeks. Fig. 3 illustrates the effect of increasing PEG concentrations on rate and extent of tobramycin release. Incorporation of 30% PEG resulted in almost complete release (>95%) within 3 days.

Table 2 indicates that the initial rapid rate of release did not differ significantly while differences were observed with the slower diffusion phase. The changes in the

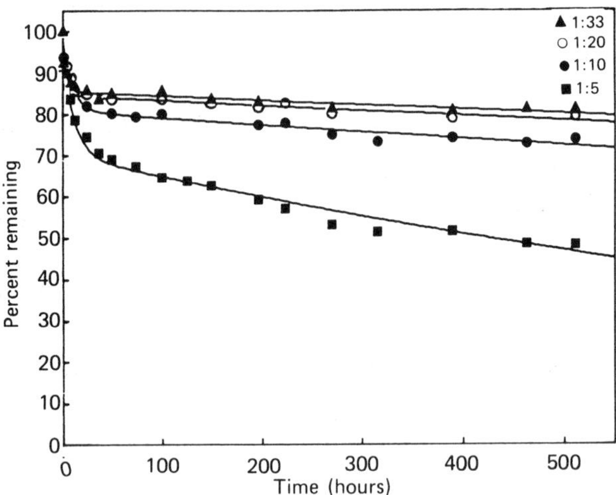

Fig. 1 — The effect of drug loading on tobramycin sulphate release profiles. The solid lines represent the lines of best fit. The symbols represent the observed values.

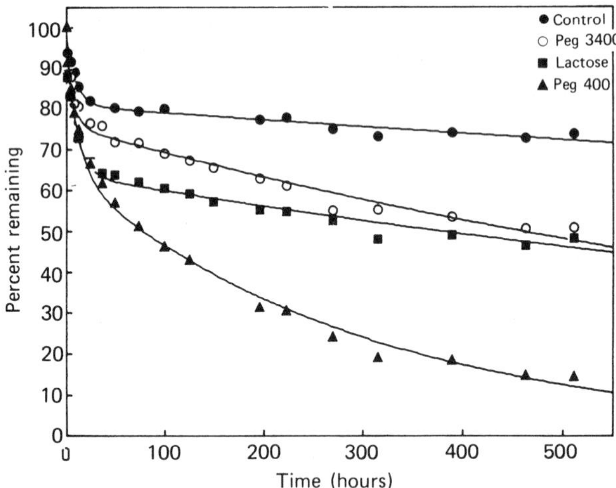

Fig. 2 — The effect of incorporation of 10% water-soluble additives on tobramycin sulphate release profiles. The solid lines represent the lines of best fit. The symbols represent the observed values.

rates and extents of drug release due to increases in drug loading and incorporation of additives can be attributed to modifications in the porosity of the implants with changes in formulation.

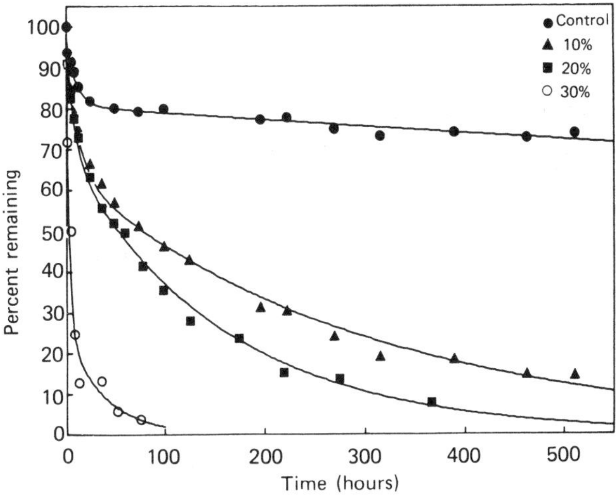

Fig. 3 — The effect of increasing levels of PEG 400 on tobramycin sulphate release profiles. The solid lines represent the lines of best fit. The symbols represent the observed values.

Studies using smaller implants of 2.9 mm diameter indicated statistically significant differences in the two rate constants (Table 2) and extent of drug released from the implant in comparison with implants of mean diameter 6.2 mm. This could be attributed to an increase in surface area per unit volume of the smaller implant.

The effect of varying dissolution volumes on the release rates from beads prepared using a 1:10 ratio of drug:carrier indicated that no statistically significant differences were observed either in the rates or in the extent of drug release, when release studies were performed using different dissolution volumes. This is to be expected since the ability of tobramycin was not a limiting factor in controlling release rate. This fact is of clinical significance since implants placed in the diseased tissue may be exposed to varying amounts of fluids.

The amount of tobramycin sulphate remaining unreleased from the PMMA implant after 1, 3 and 7 days *in vivo* is summarized in Table 3. The very low

Table 3 — Tobramycin sulphate released *in vivo* using the osteomyelitic tibia rabbit model

Day -post-implantation	Amount remaning unreleased (mg/implant)	Percentage released
0	6.140±1.080	0.00
1	5.766±0.220	6.10± 3.67
3	5.525±0.592	10.39± 8.99
7	5.640±1.258	10.57±18.33

percentage of tobramycin sulphate released *in vivo* (10.57%) after 7 days supports the *in vitro* findings (18–20% released).

Scanning electron microscopic examination before and after dissolution and *in vivo* implantation show no significant changes in surface topography for the implants prepared as they are clinically used, that is, without additives. However, distinct changes in surface characteristics and the appearance of pores are evident with the inclusion of water-soluble additives such as polyethylene glycol 400.

CONCLUSIONS

(1) The release of tobramycin sulphate from non-biodegradable, spherical PMMA implants is biphasic and can be described by biexponential linear regression analysis.
(2) Both *in vitro* and *in vivo* results indicate that drug release is incomplete and poorly controlled from implants prepared at the drug:carrier ratio used clinically.
(3) Although the release of tobramycin sulphate can be significantly improved with the addition of water-soluble additives such as polyethylene glycol 400, our current investigations are directed toward the design and development of biodegradable implants.

ACKNOWLEDGEMENTS

We gratefully acknowledge the assistance from Eli Lilly Co., for the donation of tobramycin, and Richards Medical, Howmedica and Zimmer for the donation of the bone cements used in this study. We also would like to thank Dr D. Scott for supplying the moulds.

REFERENCES

[1] C. Torholm, L. Lidgren, L. Lindberg and G. Kahlmeter, *Clin. Orthop.*, **181**, 99 (1983).
[2] D. J. Schurman, C. Trinidade, H. P. Hirshman, K. Moser, G. Kajiyama and P. Stevens, *J. Bone Joint Surg. A,* **60**, 978 (1978).
[3] R. Soto-Hall, L. Saenz, R. Tavernetti, H. E. Cabaud and T. P. Cochran, *Clin. Orthop.*, **175**, 60 (1983).
[4] H. Wahlig, E. Dingeldein, R. Bergman and K. Reuss, *J. Bone Joint Surg. B,* **60**, 270 (1978).
[5] R. H. Guy, J. Hadgraft, I. W. Kellaway and M. S. Taylor, *Int. J. Pharm.,* **11**, 199 (1982).
[6] S. Sampath and D. H. Robinson, unpublished results.
[7] C. W. Norden, *J. Infect. Dis.,* **122**, 5410 (1970).
[8] K. J. Wilson, G. Cierny, K. R. Adams and J. T. Mader., *J. Orthop. Res.,* **6**, 279 (1988).

[9] S. W. Hoff, R. H. Fitzgerald and P. J. Kelly, *J. Bone Joint Surg. A*, **63**, 798 (1981).
[10] R. A. Elson, A. E. Jephcott, D. B. Gechie and D. Verettas, *J. Bone Joint Surg. B*, **59**, 200 (1977).
[11] K. E. Marks, C. L. Nelson and E. P. Lautenschlager, *J. Bone Joint Surg. A*, **58**, 358 (1976).
[12] B. Picknell, L. Mizen and R. Sutherland, *J. Bone Joint Surg. B*, **59**, 302 (1977).
[13] J. A. Von Frauhofer, H. C. Polk, Jr., and D., Seligson, *J. Biomed. Mater. Res.*, **19**, 751 (1985).
[14] J. A. Goodell, A. B. Flick, J. C. Hebert and J. G. Howe, *Am. J. Hosp. Pharm.*, **43**, 1454 (1986).
[15] H. T. law, R. H. Fleming, M. F. X. Gilmore,. I. D. McCarthy and S. P. F. Hughes, *J. Biomed. Eng.*, **8**, 149 (1986).
[16] M. Dittgen and W. Stahlkopf, *Drug. Dev. Ind. Pharm.*, **14** (15–17) 2417 (1988).

17

Formulation of silicone matrix systems for long-term constant release of peptides

Matthais Hoth
Parmazeutische Technologie, Universität Bonn, D-Bonn, FRG
Hans P. Merkle
Eidgenössiche Technische Hochschule, Pharmazeutisches Institut, CH-Zürich, Switzerland

SUMMARY

Theoretically, release of drug through the water-filled pores of matrix systems is expected to show a square-root-of-time dependence, with a time exponent of 0.5 and hence continual declining release rates. However, there have been many research groups finding remarkable deviations.

The aim of this work was to investigate factors which lead to deviations from the $t^{1/2}$ law and may be helpful for the development of matrix systems with constant drug release. Matrices of polydimethylsiloxane (PDMS) were prepared incorporating varying amounts of different pore-building, water-soluble hydrogels. The hydrophilic model drug was Gly–Tyr.

The following factors influencing the long-term release profiles were found: (i) total matrix loading, (ii) its dissolution rate and (ii) the viscosity of the pore-building hydrogel. A proper choice of conditions lead to release profiles with time exponents up to 0.8 for at time period of several weeks.

INTRODUCTION

Long-term controlled release of drugs from inert matrices has been subject of numerous scientific investigations (e.g. refs. [1–7]). The easily manufactured release systems may be applied as subcutaneous implants in humans and for veterinary use. They are helpful in many other areas too, for instance in agriculture [8].

THEORY

As for long-term release a comparatively high drug dose is required, drug concentration in the device will in most cases far exceed matrix solubility. Theoretical considerations may therefore be reduced to suspension-type matrix systems [9,10].

Dealing with the release of a peptide, or generally hydrophilic, water-soluble drugs, drug release will occur by pore diffusion. The pores may be part of the matrix itself or they may be formed *in situ*, as drug particles are leached out by the penetrating aqueous medium [11]. Provided that (i) water penetration and drug dissolution are much faster than pore diffusion and (ii) matrix pores are only built *in situ*, while (iii) matrix diffusion be negligible, time-dependent release is described by.

$$M(t)=F[(2A-\varepsilon C_s)(D/\tau)C_s t]^{1/2} \quad (1)$$

where M is the amount of drug released, F is the surface in contact with release medium, A, the drug concentration in matrix (matrix loading), ε the porosity of the matrix, C_s the drug solubility in matrix pores, τ the tortuosity factor of matrix pores and D the diffusion coefficient of drug in matrix pores.

Unfortunately, the $t^{1/2}$ dependence described by equation (1) is inconvenient especially for long-term drug delivery as release rates decline with time. On the other hand, there are numerous publications on matrix-type release systems showing remarkable deviations from the expected $t^{1/2}$ law (Table 1). Deviations are mainly observed when water-soluble drugs are delivered. It may further be noticed that presumably most of the corresponding experiments are based on the use of PDMS as the matrix polymer. As indicated by Table 1, in many cases matrix swelling is suggested to be the reason for the unexpected release profiles. Di Colo *et al.* [15] showed that water uptake into the matrix may indeed have a strong influence on release kinetics.

MATERIALS, METHODS

The following materials were used:

Matrix polymer: PDMS (Silastic® 382 Medical Grade Elastomer, Dow Corning Corp., Midland, MI);

Matrix embedding: PDMS (Silastic® MDX-4-4210 Medical Grade Elastomer, Dow Corning Corp., Midland, MI);

Pore-building, hydrophilic excipient: hydroxyethylcellulose (HEC), viscosity grades of 2% aqueous solution 300, 6000, 30000 mPa s, (Natrosol® 250 G, H, M, Hercules BV, Den Haag, The Netherlands);

Pore building, hydrophilic excipient: bovine serum albumin (Sigma Chemical Company, St. Louis, MO) of high and low dissolution rates (the dissolution rate of the product could be reduced by special treatment);

Model drug: Gly–Tyr (Fluka AG, Buchs, Switzerland).

Table 1 — Review of publications on release of hydrophilic drugs from matrix systems, mostly showing deviations from the $t^{1/2}$ law

Drug/ excipient in matrix	Matrix polymer	Release profiles observed; interpretation	Ref.
Chloroquine diphosphate–none	PDMS[a]	Burst, than fairly constant rates (4 months)	[1]
Morphine sulphate–sodium alginate	PDMS	Second order; matrix swelling may be the reason	[12]
Different proteins	EVA[b]	Sigmoidal, biphasic or $t^{1/2}$; matrix swelling may be the reason for deviations	[13,14]
Sodium salicylate–PEG	PDMS	Sigmoidal, eventually zero order; matrix swelling is responsible	[15]
Bovine serum albumin	PDMS	Burst, than fairly constant rates (3 months)	[16]

[a] Polydimethylsiloxane.
[b] Ethylene vinyl acetate.

Drug and excipients were sieved to obtain a particle size between 45 and 90 μm. The model drug Gly–Tyr and excipient were thoroughly dispersed in Silastic® 382 plus curing agent. Dispersions were quickly transferred to a mould. After curing (24 h, 40°C), a sheet of 1.5 mm thickness was obtained; discs about 6 mm in diameter were cut. Matrices were embedded in Silastic® MDX leaving one planer surface uncovered to meet the conditions of equation (1). The concentration of Gly–Tyr was kept at 5% (w/w), whereas the concentration of excipient varied between 25% and 45% (w/w); thus matrix loading was between 30% and 50% (w/w). Release experiments were performed under sink conditions in vials containing 10 ml of isotonic phosphate buffer pH 7.4, at 37°C. The experiments lasted 3–4 weeks with the media completely exchanged evenly two to three days. On exchange of release media, matrix swelling was observed by thoroughly weighing the embedded matrices.

Release profiles were characterized by fitting the time-exponent equation (equation (2)) to the data. Equation (2), which also includes equation (1) empirically decribes release profiles of matrices deviating from equation (1). Release exponents

n greater than 0.5 indicate time-dependent variation of parameters in equation (1) which leads to a more constant drug delivery [17].

$$M(t)=at^n \tag{2}$$

where M is the amount of drug released, a a kinetic constant and n the release exponent.

In several cases, a fit of equation (2) to the data was not statistically significant, or the residuals indicated systematic deviations due to strongly curved release profiles. Then, alternatively a fit of equation (3) was tried in order to be able to describe tendencies which occur on variation of matrix composition. In all cases the first time interval was not considered, as burst effects are to be expected which are not representative for long-term drug release.

$$M(t)=m[1-\exp(-kt)] \tag{3}$$

where M is the amount of drug released, m a kinetic constant and k the release constant.

RESULTS

Matrices containing HEC

The results for matrices containing HEC as excipient are shown in Table 2 and Figs 1 and 2. Table 2 shows that only at the lowest matrix loading (30% (w/w)) could equation (2) be fitted to release data. It may further be seen that at this loading level release exponents n always yield values which exceed the value of 0.5. In one class a release exponent of 0.79 is obtained.

For higher matrix loading equation (3) obviously fits better to release data. It is expected that the curvature of release profiles and hence the tendency of the release rate to decline are too strong to be fitted to equation (2). At a matrix loading of 50% (w/w) (in one case even at 40% loading) any fit was impossible owing to rapid matrix depletion. Finally, as expected, the average release rate strongly increases at higher matrix loading. Table 2 and Fig. 2 further show the influence of excipient viscosity on matrix release: it may be seen, that increased excipient viscosity always leads to stronger declining release rates. At 30% (w/w) loading level, increased excipient viscosity leads to a marked reduction of the release exponent n. At the 40% loading level the same tendency is observed, as expressed by the release constant k which increases with excipient viscosity. In all cases, the average release rate is affected. It is strongly reduced when excipient viscosity increases. Because of rapid matrix depletion, effects could not be evaluated for 50% (w/w) matrix loading.

Matrices containing BSA

The results for matrices containing BSA are shown in Table 2 and Fig. 3. A strong influence of the excipient's dissolution rate on release kinetics may be seen. Release

Table 2 — Results of fitting parameters a, and n of equation (2) or parameters l, and m of equation (3) to release data of matrices containing HEC or BSA

Viscosity grade (m Pas)	Disolution rate	Matrix loading (% (w/w))	Parameter values			
			Equation (2)		Equation (3)	
			a	n	l	m
Matrices containing HEC						
300		30	50.1	0.792		
6000		30	25.9	0.606		
30000		30	13.2	0.556		
300		35	(147.5)	(0.652)	1417	0.067
300		40	Fast depletion of matrix			
6000		40	(122.6)	(0.647)	1206	0.063
30000		40			870	0.115
		50	At all viscosity grades, fast depletion of matrix			
Matrices containing BSA						
	High	40			1099	0.181
	High	50	Fast depletion of matrix			
	Low	30	Amounts released within tolerance of HPLC assay			
	Low	40	36.0	0.750		
	Low	50	(82.3)	(0.800)	1607	0.040

Results are not given if fits were not possible. Inferior results are given in parentheses.

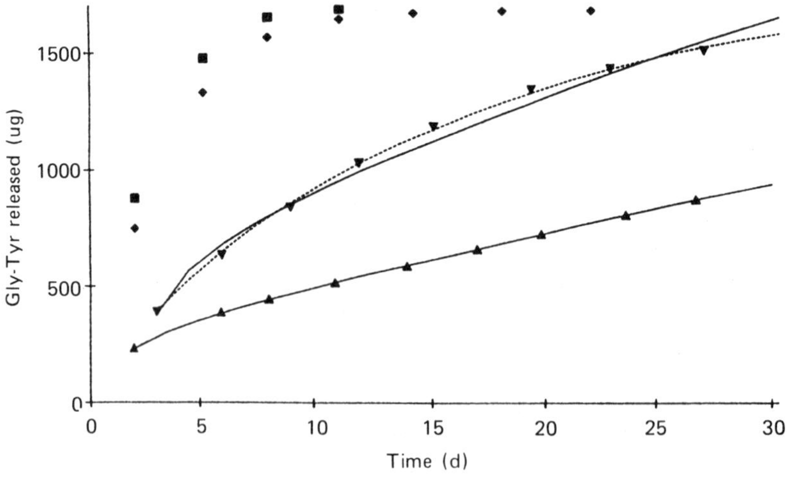

Fig. 1 — Gly–Tyr release from PDMS matrices containing HEC (viscosity grade 300 mPa s) matrix loadings (w/w): ▲, 30%; ▼, 35%; ◆, 40%, ■, 50%. ——, fit of equation (2); ---, fit of equation (3). Mean values, n=3.

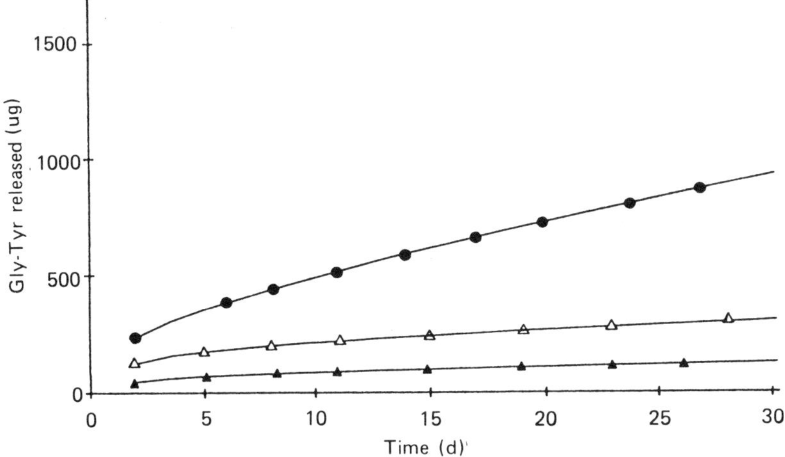

Fig. 2 — Gly–Tyr release from PDMS matrices containing HEC (matrix loading 30% (w/w)). Viscosity grades of excipient were 300 (●), 6000 (△), and 30000 (▲) mPas. ——, fit of equation (2). Mean values, $n=3$.

exponents n are obtained which are markedly higher than 0.5. However, at 50% (w/w) loading the residuals suggest small but systematic deviations from equation (2) and equation (3) is fitted better after about 2 weeks. Average release rates are strongly reduced when a slowly dissolving excipient is used.

In contrast to matrices containing (quickly dissolving) HEC, average release rates for slowly dissolving BSA are very slow even at 50% (w/w) loading; release rates for 30% matrix loading were so small that amounts released were almost within the tolerance of the HPLC assay. With quickly dissolved BSA, matrices behaved similarly to devices containing HEC.

RELEASE MECHANISM

The results show, that release profiles never followed a $t^{1/2}$ law (equation (1)). A marked influence of the excipient's viscosity grade or dissolution rate on drug release is further observed. The swelling profiles for matrices containing low-viscosity HEC or BSA are shown in Figs 4–6. The profiles show that maximum swelling is always observed in cases of quick drug depletion and bent release cures. Only in cases where maxima of swelling profiles are not observed do the corresponding release profiles show a reduced decline of release rates. The results further show that for the quickly dissolving excipient (HEC) low matrix loading is a prerequisite for fitting equation (1) and getting release exponents greater than 0.5. For slowly dissolving BSA, however, reduced decline or release rates may also be obtained at high loading levels up to 50% (w/w). Finally, a gravimetric assay of matrices shows that the residence time of excipient is markedly prolonged if matrix loading is low or if the dissolution rate of excipient is reduced (Table 3).

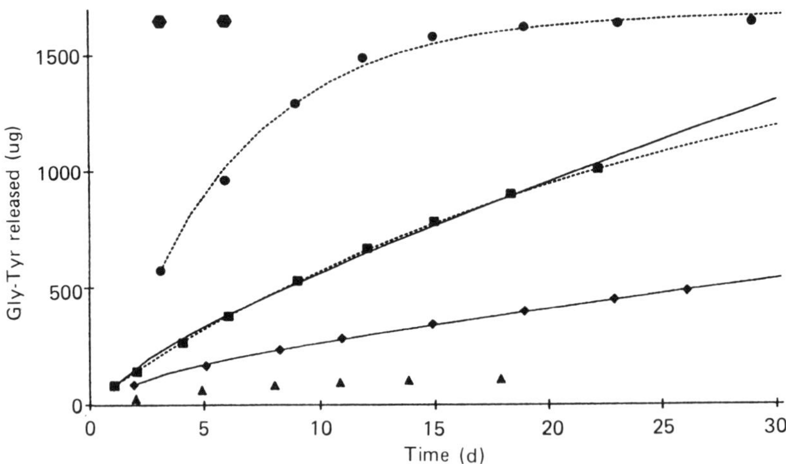

Fig. 3 — Gly–Tyr release from PDMS matrices containing BSA. Quickly dissolving BSA: matrix loadings (w/w) of 40% (●) and 50% (⬡). Slowly dissolving BSA: loadings (w/w) of 30% (▲), 40% (◆), and 50% (■). Fits of equation (2) (——) and equation (3) (- - -) are shown. Mean values, $n=3$.

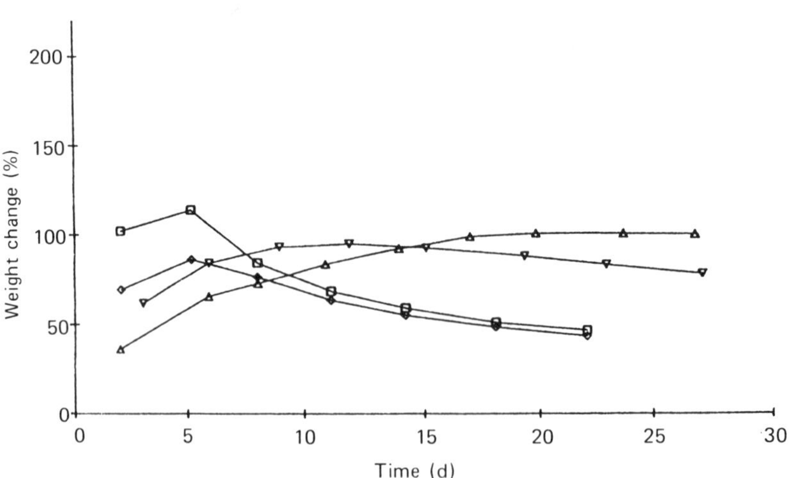

Fig. 4 — Weight change (% (w/w)) during Gly–Tyr release from PDMS matrices (matrix excipient HEC, viscosity grade 300 mPa s) for the following matrix loadings (w/w): △, 30%; ▽, 35%; ◇, 40%; □, 50%. Mean values, $n=3$.

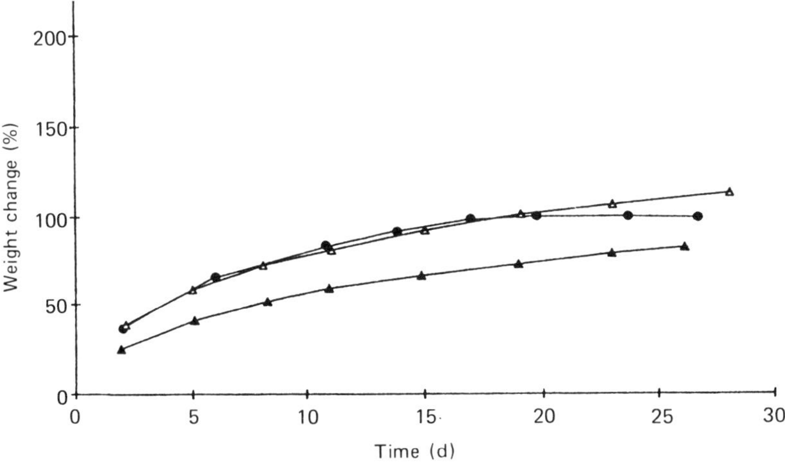

Fig. 5 — Weight change (% (w/w)) during Gly–Tyr release from PDMS matrices containing HEC (matrix loading 30% (w/w)). Viscosity grade of HEC were 300 (●), 6000 (△), and 30 000 (▲) mPa s. Mean values, $n=3$.

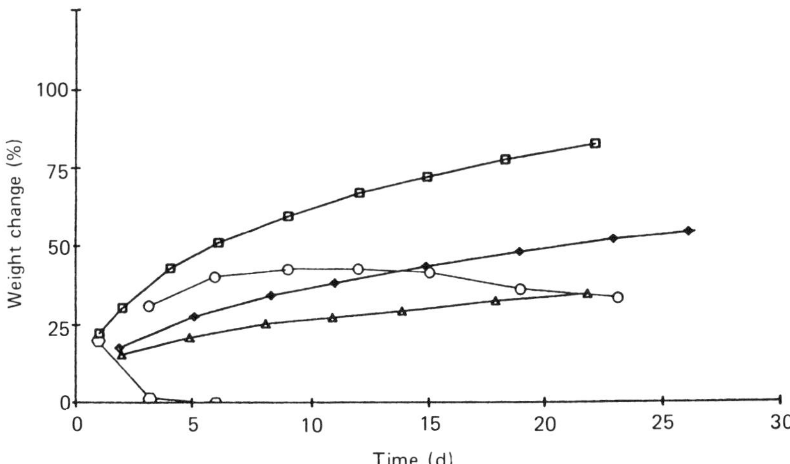

Fig. 6 — Weight change (% (w/w)) during Gly–Tyr release from PDMS matrices containing BSA. Quickly dissolving BSA: matrix loadings (w/w) of 40% (○) and 50% (⬡). Slowly dissolving BSA: Loadings (w/w) of 30% (△), 40% (◇), 50% (□). Mean values, $n=3$.

These observations suggest that a prerequisite for getting long-term drug release and release and release exponents above 0.5 is long-term retention of the excipient within the pores. Obvously, the hydrated, hydrocolloid-type excipients in the matrix pores act as diffusion medium for the drug.

In the case of a high dissolution rate of excipient and/or high matrix loading, strong initial swelling, rapid depletion of matrix excipient and consequently depletion of the elastic matrix pores occur. This should lead to curved release plots. It is

Table 3 — Residual amount of excipient and water content of remaining excipient in matrix after 16 days of release

Viscosity grade (mPa s)	Disolution rate	Matrix loading (% w/w))	Excipient after 16 days	
			Residual amount (% (w/w))	Water content (% (w/w))
HEC excipient				
300		30	92.0	82.4
6000		30	92.6	82.4
30000		30	92.3	74.4
300		40	73.9	83.4
6000		40	72.9	81.6
30000		40	73.5	85.2
BSA excipient				
	High	50	56.1	64.8
	Low	50	92.3	64.3

noteworthy that swelling maxima have no influence on release profiles; obviously, therefore, excipient is released from zones of the matrix already drug depleted.

On the other hand, when the excipient is leached out slowly, long-term swelling within the pores obviously contributes to time-dependent changes of parameters from equation (1). This may lead to release exponents exceeding the value of 0.5. The diffusion coefficient D may increase on swelling [18]; as shown in Table 2 and Fig. 2, a suitable viscosity grade is essential for convenient release profiles. Increasing porosity ε or decreasing tortuosity τ may counteract the tendency for the release rate to decline.

So, constant long-term release from matrix systems may preferably be realized under the following conditions: (i) hydrocolloids should be used as pore-forming excipients, (ii) excipients should be leached out very slowly and (iii) the matrix polymer should be elastic and permeable to water vapour in order to permit swelling and to yield homogeneous water uptake. Finally (iv) the swelling, drug-saturated excipient should be of higher osmotic activity than the surrounding medium in order to permit water uptake.

The results show that this concept is capable of long-term 'anomalous diffusion' [17]. Further optimization may lead to matrix-type release systems capable of even longer and more constant drug release.

REFERENCES

[1] J. C. Fu, A. K. Kale, and D. L. Moyer, Drug-incorporated silicone discs as sustained release capsules. I. Chloroquione diphosphate, *J. Biomed. Mater. Res.*, **7**, 79–93 (1973).

[2] Y. W. Chien, *Novel Drug Delivery Systems*, Dekker, New York, 1982.
[3] D. N. Robertson, I. Sivin, H. A. Nash, J. Braun and J. Dinh, Release rates of levonorgestrel from silastic capsules, homogeneous rods and covered rods in humans, *Contraception*, **27**, 483–495 (1983).
[4] D. S. T. Hsieh, K. Mann and Y. W. Chien, Enhanced release of drugs from silicone elastomers (I–IV), *Drug Dev. Ind. Pharm.*, **11**, 1391–1446 (1985).
[5] R. Langer, Biomaterials: new perspectives on their use in the controlled delivery of polypeptides, *Pharm. Technol.*, **10** (October), 35–37 (1985).
[6] L. R. Brown, C. L. Wei and R. Langer, *In vivo* and *in vitro* release of macromolecules from polymeric drug delivery systems, *J. Pharm. Sci.*, **72**, 1181–1185.
[7] R. Burns, G. McRae and L. M. Sanders, A one year controlled release system for the LHRH agonist RS-49947, in: *Proc. 15th Int. Symp. on Controlled Release of Bioactive Materials, Lincolnshire*, 1988.
[8] N. A. Peppas, and R. J. Haluska (eds.), *Proc. 12th Int. Symp. on Controlled Release of Bioactive Materials, Lincolnshire, IL*, 1985.
[9] T. Higuchi, Mechanism of sustained action medication, *J. Pharm. Sci.*, **52**, 1145–1149 (1963).
[10] S. J. Desai, A. P. Simonelli and W. J. Higuchi, Investigation of factors influencing release of solid drug dispersed in inert matrices I, *J. Pharm. Sci.*, **54**, 1459–1464 (1965).
[11] H. Fessi, J. P. Marty, F. Puisieux and J. T. Carstensen, The Higuchi square root equation applied to matrices with high content of soluble drug substance, *Int. J. Pharm.*, **1**, 265–274 (1978).
[12] J. W. McGinity, L. A. Hunke and A. B. Combs, Effect of water soluble carriers on morphine sulfate release from a silicone polymer, *J. Pharm. Sci.*, **68**, 662–664 (1979).
[13] R. Langer and J. Folkman, Sustained release of macromolecules from polymers, in R. J. Kostelnik (ed.), *Polymeric Delivery Systems*, Gordon and Breach, New York, 1978.
[14] R. Langer, Controlled release of macromolecules, *Chemtech*, **3** (February), 98–105 (1982).
[15] G. Di Colo, V. Campigli, V. Carelli, E. Nannipieri, M. F. Serafini and D. Vitale, Release of osmotically active drugs from silicone rubber matrices, *Farmaco, Ed. Prat.*, **39**, 377–389.
[16] D. S. T. Hsieh, C. C. Chiang, D. S. Desai, Controlled release of macromolecules from silicone elatomer, *Pharm. Technol.*, **6**, 39–49 (1985).
[17] P. Ritger and N. A. Peppas, A simple equation for description of solute release II, *J. Control. Release*, **5**, 37–42 (1987).
[18] B. W. Barry, *Dermatological Formulations*, Dekker, New York, 1983, pp. 81–85.

Index